DISABLING PERVERSIONS

FORENSIC PSYCHOTHERAPY MONOGRAPH SERIES

Series Editor: Professor Brett Kahr
Honorary Consultant: Dr Estela V. Welldon

Other titles in the Series

Violence: A Public Health Menace and a Public Health Approach
Edited by Sandra L. Bloom

Life Within Hidden Walls: Psychotherapy in Prisons
Edited by Jessica Williams Saunders

Forensic Psychotherapy and Psychopathology: Winnicottian Perspectives
Edited by Brett Kahr

Dangerous Patients: A Psychodynamic Approach to Risk Assessment and Management
Edited by Ronald Doctor

Anxiety at 35,000 Feet: An Introduction to Clinical Aerospace Psychology
Robert Bor

The Mind of the Paedophile: Psychoanalytic Perspectives
Edited by Charles W. Socarides

Violent Adolescents: Understanding the Destructive Impulse
Lynn Greenwood

Violence in Children: Understanding and Helping Those Who Harm
Edited by Rosemary Campher

Murder: A Psychotherapeutic Investigation
Edited by Ronald Doctor

Psychic Assaults and Frightened Clinicians: Countertransference in Forensic Settings
Edited by John Gordon and Gabriel Kirtchuk

Forensic Aspects of Dissociative Identity Disorder
Edited by Adah Sachs and Graeme Galton

Playing with Dynamite: A Personal Approach to the Psychoanalytic Understanding of Perversions, Violence, and Criminality
Estela V. Welldon

The Internal World of the Juvenile Sex Offender: Through a Glass Darkly then Face to Face
Timothy Keogh

DISABLING PERVERSIONS
Forensic Psychotherapy with People with Intellectual Disabilities

Alan Corbett

Forensic Psychotherapy Monograph Series

KARNAC

First published in 2014 by
Karnac Books Ltd
118 Finchley Road
London NW3 5HT

British Library Cataloguing in Publication Data

A C.I.P. for this book is available from the British Library

ISBN-13: 978-1-78220-163-2

Typeset by V Publishing Solutions Pvt Ltd., Chennai, India

Printed in Great Britain

www.karnacbooks.com

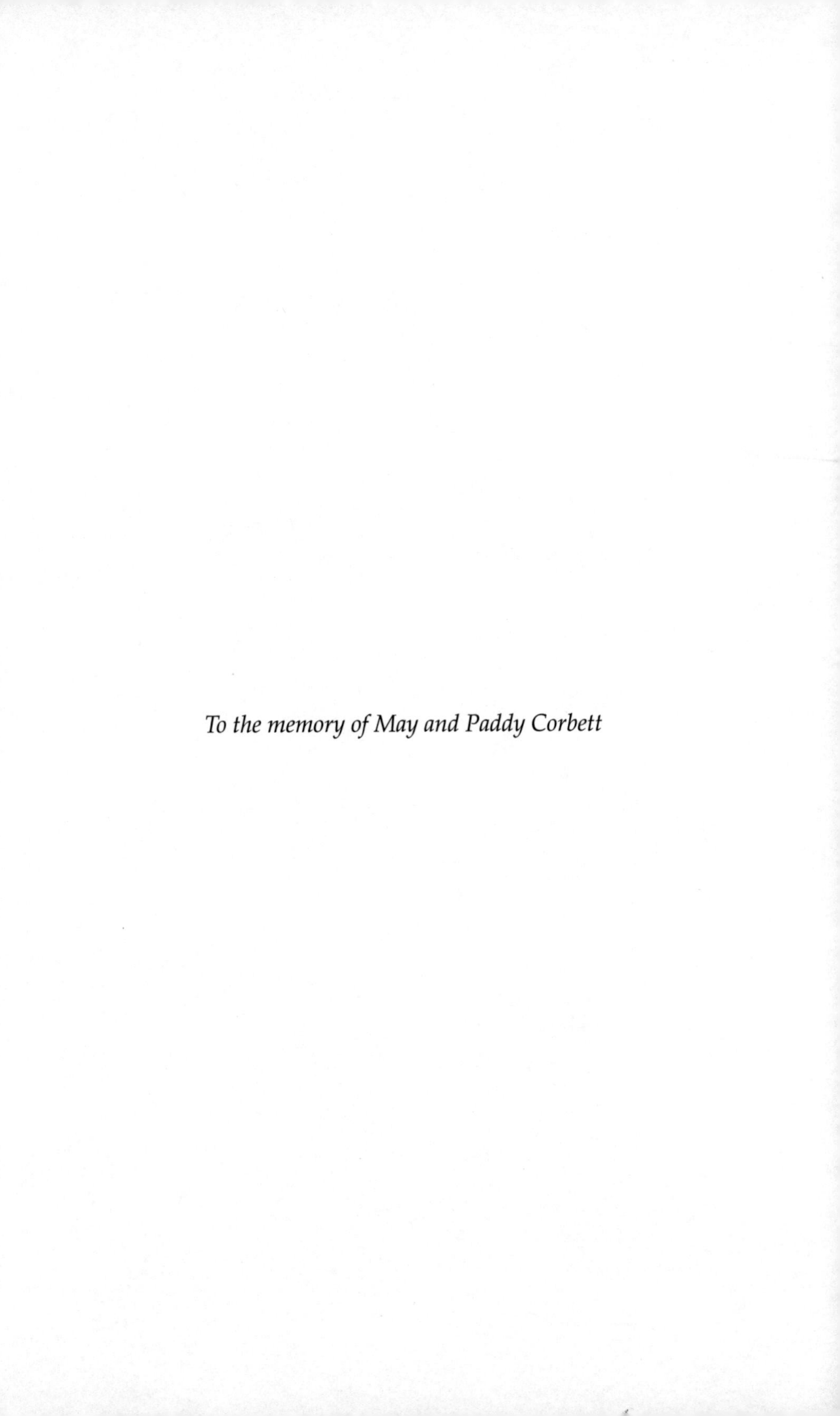

To the memory of May and Paddy Corbett

CONTENTS

ACKNOWLEDGEMENTS

As there is no specific training course on forensic disability psychotherapy, this book is the result of a hybrid of clinical experiences over the past twenty years. Foremost amongst these was my decade at Respond, which remains the UK's foremost provider of psychotherapy to children and adults with intellectual disabilities. Respond would not exist without the remarkable foresight, creativity and continuing energy of Tamsin Cottis, and this book would not have been written without her inspiration and friendship. I am grateful also to all those therapists with whom I worked in my time at Respond, and those with whom I still work as supervisor.

Respond and I were astonishingly lucky in having Valerie Sinason as our first supervisor. Valerie is the pioneer of disability therapy and, from the very early days, encouraged us all to work with the abused inside the abuser, and vice versa. I am very grateful for the courage with which she has approached therapy with those deemed unreachable by traditional psychoanalysis. Anne Alvarez took Valerie's place at Respond and was probably the only person who was able to do so. Anne continues to supervise my clinical work and I hope that this book reflects her attention to clinical detail and her ability to find humanity in the most emotionally impoverished patients. This triumvirate of incredible women whose commitment to the therapeutic needs of people with disabilities has so influenced my thinking is completed by Baroness Hollins. Sheila's commitment to parity of esteem for all has helped shape this book, and her creation of the "Books Beyond Words" series stands as a testament to her unflagging commitment to the human rights of both victims and perpetrators of abuse who have intellectual disabilities.

I was fortunate to have trained at the Portman Clinic under the guidance of Estela Welldon, and even luckier to have been supported by Estela and our colleagues at the International Association for Forensic Psychotherapy to keep the needs of patients with disabilities at the forefront of our awareness. Estela's generosity of spirit and her clarity of forensic thinking have influenced a generation of therapists. I would also like to thank Gwen Adshead, Anna Motz, Richard Curen, and other colleagues in the IAFP for taking such an inclusive view of forensic work with patients with disabilities, always ensuring it has a home and a voice. My special thanks are due to Earl Hopper, whose guidance, insight, and support have been key to my development as a therapist. His thinking about trauma in organisations and his unique understanding of group processes continue to inform all aspects of my practice.

My colleagues at the Institute of Psychotherapy and Disability have provided support and validation at those times when the work has been particularly difficult to bear. I am fortunate to have peers such as Noelle Blackman, Pat Frankish, Nigel Beail, Georgina Parkes, Nancy Sheppard, and many others in the IPD to help share the load. My thanks must also go to Georgia Lepper who supervised my doctoral thesis from which my thinking on notions of consent in the forensic narrative developed. Her insight and support were invaluable.

* * *

Finn Conlon's sculpture and Kathryn Whelan's photography for the cover of this book has been a joy to be part of, and my thanks go to them and Angelina Veiga for their generous creativity. Speaking of generosity, my particular thanks go to Brett Kahr, who has been an unflaggingly supportive editor. His belief in the concept of forensic disability therapy and his desire to see it documented in this book have made the whole endeavour possible.

This book draws upon many case examples. To protect confidentiality any information about individuals has been modified and anonymised. The aim has not been to represent particular people, but to illustrate and bring alive the deep and complex challenges involved in working psychoanalytically with forensic patients with disabilities. This extends to those examples drawn from my work as a supervisor, and I am grateful to my supervisees for teaching me so much about the harsh realities of life as a forensic disability therapist, both in the consulting room and in a variety of different institutional settings.

I would finally like to thank my partner Peter McKeown for his patience, love, and support during the writing of this book, and beyond.

ABOUT THE AUTHOR

Dr Alan Corbett is a psychoanalytic psychotherapist and supervisor. He is a trustee and member of the Institute of Psychotherapy and Disability, and member of the Guild of Psychotherapists. He has been Clinical Director of Respond, the CARI Foundation, and ICAP, is a Consultant Psychotherapist with the Clinic for Dissociative Studies and the School of Life, and teaches on a number of psychoanalytic trainings in London and Dublin.

SERIES EDITOR'S FOREWORD

Towards forensic disability psychotherapy

> *"Nemo fit fato nocens".*
> ["No one is driven to crime by fate"/"Fate makes no one guilty"].
>
> —Lucius Annaeus Seneca, *Oedipus*, first century A.C.E.

Just moments before I sat down to write my foreword to Dr Alan Corbett's wonderful new book *Disabling Perversions: Forensic Psychotherapy with People with Intellectual Disabilities*, I watched a highly disturbing news broadcast on the television. The previous day, 29 April 2014, Clayton Darrell Lockett, a thirty-eight-year-old American man, condemned to die for the kidnap, rape, and murder of nineteen-year-old Stephanie Neiman, suffered his own gruesome death in the Oklahoma State Penitentiary in McAlester, Oklahoma. After strapping Lockett to an execution table, a prison authority administered a lethal cocktail of midazolam (a benzodiazepine), vecuronium bromide (a muscle relaxant), and potassium chloride (a chemical compound, lethal in large quantities). Although the hearts of most felons will stop beating within six to twelve minutes after such a combination of drugs has entered the bloodstream, Lockett's execution did not proceed according to plan, and in spite of the deadly dosage, he remained alive for a full forty-three minutes, during which time he spoke, exhaled, twitched, and convulsed. One of the physicians on duty had to interrupt the execution in order to investigate the situation. Eventually, Clayton Lockett suffered a fatal coronary, and, thus, the convicted murderer finally died.

Clayton Lockett had committed an act of barbarism, first kidnapping the teenage Miss Neiman, then beating her, raping her with his accomplices, shooting her, and finally, burying her alive. Many would argue that such a sadistic man did not deserve to live, and that he thus merited this judicially sanctioned death. Some people may even have enjoyed the fact that Lockett writhed in pain on the execution table, experiencing such a protracted dying process. Whatever one's view, we cannot deny that Oklahoma state law "treated" a murderer by murdering him in turn. An eye for an eye …

Does the execution of a convicted criminal represent a sensible approach to crime prevention, by punishing the guilty in the hope of deterring those at risk? Or does it constitute what psychotherapists and psychoanalysts might regard as an unconscious identification with the aggressor?

Throughout much of history, human beings have dealt with offenders—whether vagrants, villains, outlaws, gangsters, hooligans, thugs, racketeers, or killers—by punishing them, often with a cruelty which exceeded the original crime, somewhat akin to the incarceration of "Jean Valjean", immortal fictional hero of Victor Hugo's *Les Misérables*, who stole bread to feed his starving family. During Elizabethan times, for instance, miscreants would be subjected to any number of tortures, whether flung into a windowless pit, or manacled to a rack, or placed in hand-crushing iron gauntlets, before being burned, hanged, disembowelled, quartered, or beheaded, or, in certain instances, even crushed to death, by a process known as the *peine forte et dure*, a form of execution sanctioned in England since at least 1275. Sometimes, after such grisly executions, the bodies of criminals would then be subjected to dissection for medical research (Rütten, 2011). Indeed, when in Act IV, Scene v, of William Shakespeare's play *The Tragedy of Hamlet, Prince of Denmark*, "Claudius", the Danish king, expounds, "And where th'offense is, let the great axe fall", he typifies quite chillingly the attitude towards perpetrators throughout most of the last millennium.

Disgusted by the cruel treatment of criminals, many humanitarians have long fought for more sensitive and more liberal approaches to imprisonment. Mental health professionals, in particular, have argued that offenders should, where necessary, be incarcerated for reasons of safety but, also, that they should be provided with psychological *treatment*, and not subjected to *punishment*.

The psychotherapeutic approach to the study of criminality began, perhaps, on 6 February 1907, when members of the Wiener Psychoanalytische Vereinigung [Vienna Psycho-Analytical Society], held a discussion on the psychology of vagrancy. During the course of the meeting, Professor Sigmund Freud, anticipating the clarion call of subsequent forensic psychotherapists, bemoaned the often horrible treatment of mentally ill offenders. According to Otto Rank, Freud's secretary at the time, the founder of psychoanalysis expressed his sorrow at the "unsinnige Behandlung dieser Leute (soweit sie Demenz zeigen) in Gefängnissen" (quoted in Nunberg & Federn, 1976, p. 101) ["nonsensical treatment of these people in prisons (in so far as they are demented)"] (quoted in Nunberg & Federn, 1962, p. 108).

The brutal treatment of criminals hardly surprised Freud, who knew only too well about the cruel underbelly of human behaviour. Indeed, late in life, Freud wrote to the German literary critic and political dissident Professor Georg Fuchs (1931), congratulating him on the publication of his book, *Wir Zuchthäusler: Errinerungen des Zellengefangenen Nr. 2911* [*We Convicts: Memories of Prisoner in Cell Number 2911*]—a critique of punition in penal institutions—based on Fuch's own incarceration. As Freud (1931a, p. x) explained, "Ich könnte zum Beispiel den Satz nicht unterschreiben, daß die Behandlung der Strafgefangenen eine Schande für unsere Kultur ist. Im Gegenteil, würde mir eine Stimme sagen: sie ist ganz in Einklang mit unserer Kultur, notwendige Äußerung der Brutalität und des Unverstandes, die die gegenwärtige Kulturmenschheit beherrschen." ["I could not, for example, subscribe to the sentence that the way prisoners are treated is a disgrace to our civilization. On the contrary, a voice would tell me: it is quite in accord with our civilization, a necessary manifestation of the brutality and the folly that dominate present civilized mankind."] (Freud, 1931b, p. 199).

Freud inspired numerous colleagues to explore the possibilities of deploying psychoanalysis in the understanding and treatment of those who had committed crimes. And throughout the 1920s and 1930s, and beyond, a range of pioneering mental health workers across the globe made useful contributions to the burgeoning field of psychoanalytical criminology.

As early as 6 March 1912, Alfred Freiherr von Winterstein addressed his colleagues in the Wiener Psychoanalytische Vereinigung on forensic matters, highlighting criminology as one of the areas ripe for the application of psychoanalysis. And many responded to this invitation. For instance, Dr Hanns Sachs, a trained lawyer and one of Freud's earliest disciples, spoke about the death penalty for offenders as an example of group sadism (Moellenhoff, 1966); and in a similar vein, the princesse Marie Bonaparte, Freud's sometime analysand, wrote years later about the cruelty of war, and, like Sachs, also objected fiercely to capital punishment. Bonaparte had studied various murderers throughout her career, from Madame Lefebvre (the former Marie Felicité Elise Lemaire) to Peter Kürten, the so-called "Vampire of Düsseldorf", to the matricidal American woman Jo Ann Baker. The French princess had even lobbied politicians in the United States of America to free the convicted robber and rapist Caryl Chessman from his sentence on Death Row in the California State Prison in San Quentin; and with assistance from psychoanalysts Dr Franz Alexander and Dr Isadore Ziferstein, the princesse Bonaparte sent not only a petition to Governor Edmund Brown of California, but also a pleading letter to President John Fitzgerald Kennedy, albeit to no avail (Bertin, 1982). Marie Bonaparte's work on this subject, *Les Faux-pas de la justice* [*The Faux-Pas of Justice*], has remained unpublished.

Others, too, made enormous contributions to this growing branch of endeavour, ranging from the Viennese psychoanalyst Dr Theodor Reik, who treated a paedophile (under the supervision of Freud himself) (Natterson, 1966), to the German psychoanalyst Dr Clara Happel (1926) who studied the nature of paederasty and genital exhibitionism (cf. Stoddart, 1923; Alexander & Staub, 1929; Chadwick, 1932; Oberndorf, 1939; Lorand, 1940). The seminal Hungarian psychoanalyst Dr Sándor Ferenczi (1922) even devoted an entire chapter on "Psychoanalyse und Kriminologie" ["Psycho-Analysis and Criminology"] in his book *Populäre Vorträge über Psychoanalyse* [*Popular Lectures on Psycho-Analysis*].

A South American physician, Dr Juan Ramón Beltrán, also practised Freudian psychology in a prison setting, offering treatment to an inmate instead of further punishment. Beltrán's work had so impressed the founder of the German psychoanalytical movement,

Dr Karl Abraham (1924a, p. 766), that he wrote to Professor Sigmund Freud with much enthusiasm, "Der Autor hat in einer Strafanstalt einen wegen Mordes Verurteilen ziemlich weitgehend und sehr verständnisvoll analysiert! So etwas muß aus Südamerika zu uns kommen!" ["In a prison the author has analysed quite deeply, and, with much understanding, a man sentenced for murder! This sort of thing has to come to us from South America!"] (Abraham, 1924b, p. 505). Beltrán's pioneering contribution may well have inspired Abraham himself to deliver three lectures on "Psychoanalytic Theory of Crime (For jurists, medical doctors and pedagogues)", at the Berliner Psychoanalytisches Institut [Berlin Psycho-Analytical Institute] during the second quarter of 1925.

Even in faraway India, the early psychoanalysts helped to pioneer forensic psychoanalysis. On 30 July 1925, Dr Girindrasekhar Bose, the founder of the Indian Psycho-Analytical Society and its first President, addressed the Calcutta Parliament on the subject of psychoanalysis and criminality. He also spoke to the Bengal Legislative Assembly on the same subject, and even taught a course on psychoanalysis and crime for the Principal Detective School in India (Hartnack, 2001). Furthermore, Bose provided expert witness testimony for the defence in a "sensational political murder case" (Banerji, 1925, p. 242), as a result of which, Indian jurists became increasingly interested in psychoanalytical ideas. Contemporaneously, on 20 August 1925, Dr Sarasilal Sarkar, a Civil Surgeon in Noakhali, Bengal, and an early member of the Indian Psycho-Analytical Society, delivered a talk to his colleagues on "Psychology of a Murderer" (Anonymous, 1926).

In Great Britain, most especially, a number of other very forward-thinking clinicians made huge contributions to the psychoanalytical study of crime and delinquency, concentrating their efforts on understanding the nature of crime (known as *criminosis*), the causes of crime (known as *crimongenesis*), and the treatment thereof. These distinguished psychoanalytical practitioners included Dr Montague David Eder, one of the first—if not *the* first—men to practice psychoanalysis in the United Kingdom. Eder had worked for a time at the Clinic for Juvenile Delinquents (Jones, 1936), and he would ultimately contribute to the development of the Institute for the Scientific Treatment of Delinquency (later renamed the Institute for the Study and Treatment of Delinquency) along with other colleagues such as Dr Marjorie Franklin, Dr Edward Glover (1956), Dr Ethilda Budgett-Meakin Herford

(Payne, 1957), Dr Grace Pailthorpe, and Dr Melitta Schmideberg (who also had a longstanding involvement in the Howard League for Penal Reform).

Dr Maurice Hamblin Smith, an early Associate Member of the British Psycho-Analytical Society, made particularly valiant contributions to the profession. A prison psychiatrist with a longstanding interest in Freudianism, Smith held the post of Medical Officer at H. M. Prison Winson Green in Birmingham from 1920 to 1933; and throughout his distinguished career, he advocated treatment for offenders rather than punishment, earnestly hoping to turn prisons into hospitals (e.g., Smith, 1924). And Dr Cyril Wilson, another early British psychoanalyst, worked at the Broadmoor Criminal Lunatic Asylum (Winnicott, 1958), while other analysts, notably Dr John Bowlby (1944a, 1944b), Dr Kate Friedlander (1947), and Dr Donald Winnicott (1935, 1943, 1956, 1962–1963, 1966, 1968, n.d.; cp. Kahr, 2001) applied psychoanalytical insights to the fields of child and adolescent psychiatry, contributing mightily to the understanding of juvenile delinquency. Even the Hungarian-born psychoanalyst Dr Michael Balint (1951), although not primarily a forensic mental health specialist, discoursed upon the cruelty of punishing offender patients.

In the decades which have followed, the field of forensic psychotherapy (sometimes referred to as forensic psychoanalysis) has become increasingly potent and impactful. In 1991, under the inspiring leadership of Dr Estela Welldon, colleagues from all over the world congregated at St. Bartholomew's Hospital in London for the inaugural conference of the International Association for Forensic Psychotherapy, an organisation which continues to flourish to this day, promoting education, training, treatment, and research into the ways in which those who commit crimes do so because of early traumatic experiences, which can often be ameliorated through compassionate psychotherapeutic intervention.

In spite of the growth of forensic psychotherapy, one group of offender patients has remained very poorly served by mental health professionals, namely, those who struggle with disabilities—whether physical or intellectual in nature. When I entered the mental health field during the mid-1970s, we referred to these individuals as suffering from mental retardation, and later, from mental handicap. By the 1990s, we had begun to use the phrase learning disability or learning difficulty. And more recently, the term of preference has become intellectual disability. No doubt it will change again in due course.

Disabled individuals, often thought to be "stupid", and, hence, deprived of basic literacy training, seemed to be poor candidates for Freud's "talking cure"; and many psychotherapists and psychoanalysts thus subscribed to the notion that disabled and handicapped people could not be treated because of their inability to verbalise their free associations and fantasies. A few isolated practitioners, however, did explore the possibility of using psychotherapeutic approaches with patients who had little or no formal linguistic capabilities; and here one must applaud the pioneering efforts of practitioners such as Dr Leon Pierce Clark, an early American psychoanalyst, whose book *The Nature and Treatment of Amentia: Psychoanalysis and Mental Arrest in Relation to the Science of Intelligence*, written with various colleagues (Clark, Uniker, Cushing, Rourke, & Cairns, 1933), proved groundbreaking, but alas, the work of Clark has come to be almost completely forgotten (cf. O'Driscoll, 1999, 2000, 2009). Since that time, many other noted clinicians have contributed greatly to the development of psychoanalytical and psychotherapeutic work with the disabled, notably Dr Pat Frankish, Professor the Baroness Hollins [Sheila Hollins] (Hollins, 1990a, 1990b, 1997; Hollins & Sinason, 2000), Madame Maud Mannoni (1964a, 1964b), Dr Valerie Sinason (1986, 1990, 1991, 1992, 1993, 1999, 2010), and others too numerous to mention (e.g., Grzesiak & Hicock, 1994; De Groef & Heinemann, 1999; Blackman, 2003; Wilson, 2003; Cottis, 2009b; Curen, 2009). But, in spite of the growing literature on the field we now refer to as that of disability psychotherapy (Kahr, 2000a, 2000b, 2000c, 2000d), and in spite of the copious activities of the Institute of Psychotherapy and Disability, founded in 1999, very few workers have endeavoured to provide psychoanalytical treatment for those intellectually and physically disabled patients who also commit crimes or who may be at risk of doing so. In other words, until recently, we have lacked a field of what we might call *forensic disability psychotherapy*.

Fortunately, Dr Alan Corbett has worked at the cutting edge of this vital branch of mental health practice for more than twenty-five years, and, during this time, he has distinguished himself as a leader in our field, becoming a much-admired and invaluable presence in our community. I first met Alan round about 1992 when I visited the organisation that he had helped to found—Respond—then located, I believe, somewhere in the depths of South London, and situated now, more conveniently, just a stone's throw from Euston Station in Central

London. With little funding and little professional support from the wider mental health community, Alan Corbett and a small team of comrades helped to transform Respond from a fledgling project into one of the most durable and highly regarded psychological services in the disability field.

At the outset, Respond provided psychotherapeutic interventions for learning disabled men and women who had suffered gross forms of physical abuse and sexual abuse; and hence, its client group could be described predominantly as survivors (e.g., Corbett, Cottis, & Morris, 1996). But it soon became increasingly clear that some of the disabled clients who attended Respond not only suffered abuse at the hands of others, but could also perpetrate acts of abuse, even criminality, themselves. This recognition proved most unpopular at the time, as many people could not tolerate the idea that an abused person might also be an abuser.

Throughout the 1990s, Alan became increasingly expert in the diagnosis and treatment of disabled patients, specialising in working with those with forensic complications; and when I had the privilege of becoming a Trustee of Respond in 1996, I had a unique opportunity over the next few years to watch Alan's work develop in a solid, creative, and compassionate manner. He really led the vanguard, introducing forensic disability psychotherapy at a time when few other people had either the interest or the aptitude to do so.

I had long hoped that Dr Corbett would write a textbook on forensic disability psychotherapy for the Karnac Books Forensic Psychotherapy Monograph Series, and it pleased me greatly when he submitted his elegant and groundbreaking typescript, written with such warmth and with such clarity. His evocatively-entitled contribution, *Disabling Perversions: Forensic Psychotherapy with People with Intellectual Disabilities*—his first solo-authored book—marks Alan's arrival as a figure of great stature in our field. Throughout the work, Corbett has provided us with a remarkably comprehensive map of the nature of psychotherapeutic work with the forensically disabled; and he does so with tremendous sensitivity and insight, always foregrounding the dignity of his clients, irrespective of their offences.

Alan's contribution stands as a solid piece of work, which sits comfortably in the long historical trajectory that I have outlined in the preceding pages, and in this respect, his work builds upon the original clinical researches of Sigmund Freud, Edward Glover, Donald

Winnicott, John Bowlby, Estela Welldon, Valerie Sinason, and others. But Alan has made important new strides not only by integrating the various strands of his forensic ancestors but also through his own very personal amalgam of classical psychoanalytical theory, modern relational praxis, attachment-based psychoanalysis, forensic psychology, as well as his extensive professional clinical experiences, all filtered through the lens of his sturdy, reliable, considerate, intelligent, and deeply feeling personality. In this respect, he has really helped to launch forensic disability psychotherapy as a proper speciality, which, I feel confident, will grow and grow in scope and influence in the decades to come. And I have every expectation that more books will follow from this important author.

As a Series Editor, I have the task of commissioning manuscripts, and then guiding the authors from first conception to final product. Generally, mental health professionals have little time or talent for good writing, and I often find myself in receipt of a draft that, I fear, would hardly impress a panel of literary judges. Indeed, many mental health manuscripts arrive on my desk in a somewhat disordered and plodding state. But Alan's manuscript, by contrast—so thoughtfully reasoned and so lovingly prepared—came to me in such perfect order that neither I, nor the proofreader at Karnac Books, had very much "tidying up" work to undertake. The care with which Dr Corbett completed and submitted his manuscript reflects, I believe, the care with which he works with patients in the consulting room. We count ourselves fortunate to have Dr Corbett as a member of our profession.

Disabling Perversions: Forensic Psychotherapy with People with Intellectual Disabilities stands proudly in the history of forensic psychotherapeutic work, as well as alongside the thirteen volumes published previously in this series. Our growing library of forensic psychotherapy books remains a testament to the innovative way in which contemporary mental health workers have expanded upon the work of our forefathers and foremothers to create a compassionate, considered approach to the care of psychologically troubled offenders. In doing so, forensic mental health workers have made, and will continue to make, a vital contribution to the understanding of interpersonal violence, and to its humane treatment, and, we hope, ultimately, to its very prevention. I congratulate Dr Alan Corbett on his work, and I know that the ideas contained herein will have a rich afterlife and will be used engagingly by colleagues for years to come.

I began this foreword by referring to the tragic case of the American murderer Clayton Darrell Lockett who, I suspect, may have struggled with intellectual disabilities, as well as with a profound uncontrollable rage, which resulted in a series of rapes and in a brutal death, followed by his own botched execution. According to news reports, Lockett had experienced abandonment, physical abuse, and sexual abuse by his primary caretakers during his early childhood, a background far too familiar to those of our disabled offender patients. If only the State of Oklahoma had a forensic disability psychotherapist like Alan Corbett on staff, helping this tragic man to transform his murderous deeds into murderous words, who knows just how many lives might be saved.

Professor Brett Kahr
Series Editor,
Forensic Psychotherapy Monograph Series
London

CHAPTER ONE

Disabling perversion: building a theory of forensic disability therapy

A note on language

Throughout this book I use the term "intellectual disability" rather than "learning disability" in the knowledge that within the coming decade another more "correct" term will be coined and "intellectual disability" will come to feel as anachronistic and offensive as mental handicap, spastic and idiot have come to sound to modern ears. Valerie Sinason has written of "words brought in to replace the verbal bed linen when a particular word feels too raw, too near a disturbing experience" (1992, pp. 39–40) and her beautifully crafted metaphor also touches on current sensitivities about the use of the word perversion. Welldon (1996a) writes that perversion is an accepted clinical condition in which the person afflicted does not feel free to obtain sexual genital gratification through intimate contact with another person. Instead he or she feels 'taken over' by a compulsive activity which is subjectively experienced as inexplicable and 'bizarre', but provides a release of unbearable and increasing sexual anxiety. This activity usually involves an unconscious desire to harm others or him or herself. In this usage perversion is a technical, psychoanalytic term, and carries no moral connotations (p. 273). I agree with this, just as I prefer to use "patient" rather than "client", as the latter word seems to commodify the therapeutic process, and seeks to deny the presence of illness at the core of forensic enactment.

It has been a challenge to decide how to describe those I am writing about in this book—people with intellectual disabilities who have perpetrated acts of abuse, or are at risk of doing so. I have decided upon "forensic disability patient" as a less unwieldy shorthand, and have also tended to use "he" rather than "she" when describing my patients, unless it is clear that the patient is female. I do not want this to be misread as a denial of the prevalence of women who carry out acts of abuse—far from it. The artificial divide between male abusers and female victims is a denial of the capacity of all forensic patients to act out their pain as much as act it in, regardless of gender.

I begin by thinking about language as I now realise, looking back on my 20 years of experience with forensic disability patients, that I began working with them before knowing that was what they were, let alone what I should call them. After some years working in various care homes with young people and adults with intellectual disabilities, I managed an employment service for people with intellectual disabilities in South London in the early 1990s, providing advice and information, as well as counselling. Almost inevitably, most of the referrals concerned unemployment rather than employment, with clients needing to talk about the agony of never being allowed to be part of the workforce. It did not take long in the job for me to concur with Freud's dictum that mental health depends upon the ability to love and to work, as so few of the clients I saw seemed to have had experiences of one, let alone both. I was shaken to discover that most of them had experienced abuse at some point in their lives. All the men who had had a job had lost it because of some form of sexual enactment. This included men being fired from stacking shelves in Sainsbury's and Tesco because of staring at women customers, stalking customers with babies or exposing their genitals to members of the public. While most of the men wanted to explore in their sessions with me how they could go about getting their jobs back, I found myself increasingly interested in why so many of these men were acting out sexually and, more crucially—what it was they were trying to act out. Which is what, in part, this book is attempting to answer.

The early 1990s saw a number of important changes that led to the development of forensic disability therapy. My work with the men described above soon found a home in the newly born Respond, the

UK's first psychotherapy clinic dealing exclusively with sexual abuse in the lives of people with intellectual disabilities, from where I, along with a group of colleagues, began to develop a strand of forensic services, transforming Respond from a "survivors"-only clinic to one that worked in a more integrated way with the abused, abusing, and those who were both (Corbett, 1996). The development was aided immeasurably by our clinical supervisor Valerie Sinason, who was, at the time, running a pioneering forensic group for men with intellectual disabilities with Professor Sheila Hollins. The sensitivity and bravery with which both women conducted this group was a source of inspiration to all those that worked with them. I was then fortunate enough to study forensic psychotherapy at the Portman Clinic during Estela Welldon's "Golden Decade" (Welldon, 2011) where the wish to apply psychoanalytic thinking to the perversions of patients with disabilities was, in stark contrast to other training institutes, not merely tolerated, but encouraged. While the capacity to consider the therapeutic needs of forensic patients with disabilities still has some way to go, it has travelled an enormous distance in a relatively short space of time.

To understand the development of forensic disability, we need to look first at the history of disability therapy, the birth of which can be traced to the case of the "Wild Boy of Aveyron" (Seguin, 1856). The "Wild Boy" was a French feral child who was found in 1800 after apparently spending the majority of his childhood alone in the woods. Upon his discovery, his case was taken up by a young physician, Jean Marc Gaspard Itard, who worked with the boy for five years and gave him his name, Victor. Itard broke new ground in the education of the developmentally delayed, positing what we would now understand to be a therapeutically oriented set of interventions, in stark contrast to the prevailing strict utilitarianism of the time.

Freud stated that "a certain measure of natural intelligence" was required of patients entering psychoanalysis (Freud, 1905e). He also, of course, said that psychoanalysis was not suitable for those over fifty. He wrote this when he was 49, making me wonder whether he was wishing to pull up the ladder behind him and, in doing so, created an artificial arbiter of who could benefit from analysis and who could not. Just as this may have been a defensive reaction to his own ageing process, I wonder if Freud's wish to restrict psychoanalysis to "the intelligent" was linked to a more primal fear that disability is somehow contagious. Being in the presence of someone with clear pockets of "stupidity" may evoke too much anxiety about how vulnerable our own minds are, touching on the terror we hold in our unconscious about losing our capacity to think. The most significant dissenter from Freud's view was Leon Pierce Clark, who is known today, if at all, for his work on epilepsy (1918, 1920, 1926), but who also made a major contribution to an analytic understanding of intellectual disability (1933). O'Driscoll (2009) has suggested that Pierce Clark's early death prevented a dissemination of psychotherapeutic theorising in the treatment of patients with intellectual disabilities, an idea that holds weight when one examines the relative dearth of clinical writing on intellectual disability throughout most of the twentieth century (Bender, 1993).

It should be noted that the world of art and other creative therapies worked with patients with intellectual disabilities when few others did, although little has been recorded of these decades of work. The long silence began to be broken in the 1980s and 90s, particularly by Symington in his pivotal paper "Countertransference with mentally handicapped clients" (1992) in which he considered the countertransference reactions of members of the Mental Handicap Workshop at the Tavistock Clinic. Symington encouraged his colleagues to reflect on why they tended to dress down on those days when they were seeing patients with disabilities, or why it was unthinkable that they should ever be late for any patient other than one with a disability. Symington highlighted the importance of the analytic holding and tolerating of hatred towards disabled patients and in this paper links his colleagues' unconscious underlying levels of contempt for patients with disabilities with wider historical enactments, such as the eugenics movement, the murderous intent of the Nazi party, and on a wider stage, the animal kingdom, in which the flock of birds tends to attack and kill the bird within their flock that is wounded.

Building upon Symington's developments, no one has done more than Valerie Sinason to place disability therapy into the psychoanalytic canon. Her concepts of the handicapped smile (Sinason, 1992) and the secondary handicap (Sinason, 1986) continue to inform the work of contemporary clinicians, and she has been instrumental in daring to think and write about people with disabilities not just as victims, but as abusers too. Her work inspired a wider range of clinicians to theorise on the possibilities of working psychotherapeutically with this population (Waitman & Conboy-Hill, 1992; De Groef & Heinemann, 1999) while also encouraging the building of a solid research base into the work (Beail, 1998; Beail, Warden, Morsley & Newman, 2005; Buckley, Newman, Kellett & Beail, 2006; Beail, Kellett, Newman & Warden, 2007). Her influence can also be seen in the more recent documenting of psychoanalytic approaches in working with both survivors and perpetrators of sexual abuse (Cottis, 2009a). Sinason has cemented her position as one of the pioneers of forensic disability therapy—a specialisation of a specialisation that has its roots in psychoanalytic thinking while also being open to a wide range of theoretical perspectives. The growth and development of interest in disability therapy has been cemented by the formation of the Institute of Psychotherapy and Disability, the first psychotherapy organisation working exclusively with disability to be recognised as a listing organisation by the United Kingdom Council for Psychotherapy (UKCP).

Alongside this growth of interest in working psychodynamically with patients with intellectual disabilities, the 1990s saw a realisation of the disproportionately high incidence of victims of sexual abuse who had disabilities. In the US Sobsey (1994) calculated that people with disabilities (including physical and intellectual) were four times more likely to be sexually abused than people without. In the UK it was reported that each year would see approximately 1,400 cases where sexual abuse is known to have happened, and where the victim has an intellectual disability (Brown, Stein & Turk, 1995). This latter research also contained an uncomfortable truth, that of those who had sexually abused people with intellectual disabilities, forty-one per cent were themselves disabled. It is important not to forget the impact this data had in the social care world. People had struggled to think about people with intellectual disabilities as being victims of sexual abuse. Disability is seen and experienced as antithetical to desire, making it hard to process the fact of the abuser seeking sexual gratification from someone previously thought of as ugly, unwanted and sexless. Harder still, to think of the abuser as being someone previously thought of as lacking in sexual desire, lacking both power and the intelligence needed to abuse another.

* * *

"Dennis" was referred to me for an assessment of the risk of sexual offending he posed. His mother, "Sheila", was referred to social services shortly before Dennis's birth because of concerns about her drug use. His father's identity remains unknown. Sheila disengaged from services following Dennis's birth. His moderate intellectual disability revealed itself over the course of his first three years of life, and it is reported that his four older brothers and sisters had all been diagnosed with intellectual disabilities. Over the course of Dennis's first year of life, Sheila's drug taking escalated and she began selling drugs from the family home. It is thought that Dennis witnessed his mother having sex with a number of her customers. It was reported that violent fights often erupted in the house, and Dennis was eventually placed in the care of his maternal grandmother at the age of four following an incident at home in which knives were brandished in his presence. He exhibited signs of deprivation and malnutrition, with a series of infected cuts around his body which required intensive treatment. Dennis's grandmother died when he was seven, at which point he returned to the care of his mother. Three months later, following a prolonged period of Sheila abusing drugs, he was put into the care of social services.

At the age of ten he was placed in foster care. This lasted a week, after which he was placed with another family, with whom he lived for a year. In both homes he exhibited aggressive and destructive behaviour, smeared faeces over walls and maltreated family pets. In his third placement the thirteen-year-old Dennis was found to have digitally penetrated his foster carers' eight-year-old daughter. He was then placed in a care home. His schooling was sporadic, with an ongoing series of suspensions and expulsions stemming from his propensity to stalk girls and talk to peers and teachers about his wish to rape particular children. Despite a high level of supervision and monitoring, he sexually assaulted a number of girls in his school, using excessive levels of violence and coercion.

I first met Dennis when he was 19, at which point he had a long history of self-harm. His mother had just died of a heroin overdose, and he had recently been found in the bedroom of a fifteen-year-old female resident of his care home. His team reported being at the end of the road with him, with the only hope lying in an assessment that might help another team to manage his risk of offending. Dennis himself oscillated between a swaggering bravado and an almost catatonic numbness. His level of disability appeared far higher than his IQ would suggest, and I felt as if I was in the presence of a kind of living void. Any words I used to try to construct some rudimentary kind of relationship with him were blanked out or batted away impatiently, as if words were too much for him and had to be rejected so he could focus on his primary state of numbness.

I felt very acutely the team's despondency, and their sense of failure. I wondered what, if anything, my assessment might be able to uncover, given Dennis's clear reluctance to engage with me, or with the assessment. I was able, however, to access something to dilute the sense of hopelessness. I found myself interested in Dennis's narrative. He was a young man who was hard to like, but it did seem at least possible to be interested in him. Over the course of the three-month assessment, it was this, more than any empathy, unconditional regard or basic attachment that enabled us to work together and eventually construct a clearer picture of his offending, and of his history.

The core complex

Dennis personified aspects of the core complex (Glasser, 1979), a theory that seeks to contextualise the forensic patient's perverse actions in early object relations. Glasser understood fears of annihilation and intimacy to have originated from early deprivation and neglect, and recorded the playing out of this psychopathology in adult life in the forensic patient's manic oscillation between closeness with and distance from others. The core of the complex is a fear of intimacy, a need to keep the object of sexual desire at bay, and to treat it sadistically. The forensic patient is saturated with thin-skinned narcissism (Rosenfeld, 1987), stemming from the infantile experience of the mother as being potentially overwhelming and destructive. So he has a seemingly unsolvable dilemma. He has a "deep-seated and pervasive longing for an intense and most intimate closeness to another person, amounting to a "merging", a "state of oneness", "a blissful union" (Glasser, 1979, p. 278), and yet he cannot bear the intimacy of what he wants. It has then to be retreated from, or destroyed.

The forensic disability patient is particularly vulnerable to acting out when faced with anxiety. Welldon's circular motion of perversion (Welldon, 1996a) posits sexual anxiety as coming from the conflict between the id and the superego, and locates anxiety as being the motor of sexual perversion. There is an interplay between this sexual form of anxiety and the anxiety embedded in the psychic structure of many patients with intellectual disabilities. This latter anxiety gains sustenance from the superego being brutalised by the social view of disability as being less than, the personification of damage, and the representation of all that society, and those within it, wish to disavow and turn away from. It is inordinately difficult for a child with an intellectual disability to avoid contact with the harsh and punitive brands of hatred projected into him by the world. Without wishing to pathologise disability, but while wishing equally to think about why so few patients I have worked with have possessed a healthy relationship between ego, id, and superego, I have concluded that the profoundly low levels of self-esteem, agency and psychic integrity felt by people with intellectual disabilities stem more from all that is projected into them from birth (and beyond) than from the actual fact of their low IQ.

In seeking to understand and work with Dennis's narrative, we have to assume a position of healthy dissociation, without which we could be driven mad by the barbarity of his childhood. In reading the initial referral letter, I had found myself blanking out crucial lines of information, in an attempt to dilute the agony of what I was learning. I noticed that his team also tended to do this when talking about him, so that key parts of his childhood were subtly and unconsciously edited out. Eventually I was able to find a way of letting this most horrific information into my mind without dissociating or denying, something Dennis was unable to do, either at the time or in retrospect. In his acts of sexual abuse, he was seeking to calm and subdue intense feelings of annihilation anxiety (Freud, 1926d). To stay with and think about the deprived and abused attachment to his mother was impossible for him to do as it threatened to sink him in depression. Better then to act out anxieties in sexual, life-affirming ways than to be deadened by them. He also possessed something that Glasser identifies as being key to our understanding of the forensic patient: a pathological narcissism that allowed him to turn girls into sexual objects—receptacles and containers for his desires.

In assessing Dennis it was clear that power rather than sex formed the motor for his sexual enactments. He tended to abuse others when it became too much for him to deal with how powerless he himself felt. He needed to project his powerlessness into his victims, relieving himself of feelings he lacked the ego strength to process. The only way Dennis could stop feeling as if he was being annihilated was to pass on his powerlessness to his victims. He also displayed many aspects of Welldon's diagnosis of perversion (2011), including compulsion and repetition, part-object relating and dehumanisation, all of which cathected with the issue that required most attention in his treatment—his manic defence against depression. This is a key notion in forensic psychotherapy: the inability of the patient to think about the traumata of their lives, and the need to construct manic defences to prevent any trauma from leaking into their emotional world. In considering what kind of treatment might most help Dennis, I had to think carefully about the dangers of deconstructing his defences. However dysfunctional and dangerous they were, they were familiar to him, and served to stem the imagined tide of grief that could flood him were he to get in touch with the various pains of his childhood. As will be demonstrated throughout the following chapters, in forensic work with patients with disabilities we face complex choices about how quickly we start to pick away at the protective bandages our patients have wrapped around their internal wounds.

The three secrets

Dennis's perversion may also be understood as stemming from a fundamental failure to deal with what Hollins and Grimmer (1988) call the "three secrets" of intellectual disability: dependency, sexuality, and death. These "secrets" may be seen to derive from Money-Kyrle's (1968) identification of the basic facts that need to be mastered in the cognitive development of each individual: the feeding breast, parents in creative coitus, and death. These facts of life are problematic for us all to process, of course, but I have found that my forensic disability patients have an unusually high aversion to thinking about these key areas of their life, often abusing others to escape from the painful complexities of each. Dependency for Dennis was particularly fraught, given the traumatogenic nature of his primary attachment to his mother. This cataclysmic failure of maternal containment removed the possibility of the internalisation of a good object, providing instead the conditions for an internal world riven with uncertainty and terror. The object on whom the infant Dennis should have been able to rely for consistency, safety, and holding represented instead chaos, danger, and abandonment—the prerequisites for attachment disorders that are, at best, insecure, at worst, chaotic (Solomon & George, 2011).

Many forensic disability patients live in a state of suspended childhood, their bodies growing far beyond the confines of their minds, viewed by the world as existing in a strange limbo between infancy and maturity. Time and its passing have a variety of different meanings in the world of disability and patients are sometimes robbed of the necessary developmental transitions they need to gain a fully integrated sense of self. What Piaget (1960, 1964, 1981) considered to be a series of invariant developmental stages that successively lead the child to construct a mental representation of the world will be far less applicable to the child with intellectual disabilities. The movement from one developmental stage to the next allows us not only to learn to deal with the loss of the stage we are leaving, it also enables us to deal with the fear of the stage we are about to enter. A child's sense of himself is inevitably affected also by the difficulty, common in children with intellectual disabilities, of being able to separate and then individuate from his mother (Mahler, 1971).

For forensic disability patients, the notion of dependency is inextricably bound up with disability. The baby's internalisation of the good enough mother (Winnicott, 1965b) is largely dependent on the mother's capacity to process trauma, either intrapsychically, or inter-relationally (i.e., with the help and support of the father, or other carers). Without adequate antenatal and postnatal support, it is difficult for the birth of the disabled baby to be anything other than a trauma. The narcissistic wound inflicted by the birth of the unhoped for baby is both an internal and external phenomenon. The mother not knowing where she ends and her baby begins—the "damaged" baby representing the damaged and damaging aspects of herself (akin to Wolfensberger's (1987) notion of sex leading to the birth of a disabled baby as being "death-making" rather than life-giving)—colliding with society's hatred of disability, the disabled baby as fundamentally and profoundly inferior. This conflation of the mother's fantasy of herself as someone damaging giving birth to someone damaged with society's need to relegate those with disabilities to its margins constitutes an individual and collective trauma that is inevitably projected into the baby.

Dennis's view of himself (in other words, his ego, or self) has not just been attacked by the failure of his mother to provide him with a membrane with which to protect himself against the struggles of daily life. It had also been diluted by a collective process of projective identification in which society's disavowed hatred of difference becomes located in the disabled baby, the embodiment of those disabled parts of all of us we cannot bear to think about. Dennis's childhood may be read as a story of failed dependency in which his disability has been experienced both by him and by others as a kind of grenade, primed in his mother's womb and detonated at birth.

It is in the domain of sexuality that we can see another conflation of Dennis's internal and external worlds, combining to form a matrix in which sexuality has become entangled with associations of damage, overlapping with the difficulties inherent in the first secret, that of dependency. The societal view of sexuality in the lives of people with disabilities is deeply ambivalent, with a historical locating of the subject with disabilities at polarised ends of a spectrum—either a neutered, eternal child living without any sexual feelings, or a predatory, sexual animal from whom society needs protecting. Given the boundarilessness of Dennis's early environment, it is difficult to see how he could have internalised any normal, healthy notions of sexuality as being a creative, reciprocal, and relational phenomenon. Dennis witnessing his mother engaging in sex with a number of men exposed him to a set of chaotic primal scenes he was unequipped to process. One consequence of this was Dennis's inability to have a "whole relationship"; perverse part-object relating being the best he could manage, involving, in his case, a further dehumanisation of the part-object.

Girls were not subjects, or potential people, to him. They were not even objects. They were part-objects whose presence as potential human beings was suffocated by Dennis's propensity to privilege his desires and feelings over those of anyone else. We can best understand this as a form of malignant narcissism. Weigert (1967) describes this as a regressive state involving denial and a distortion of reality, while Keogh (2011) views it as a psychic structure that underlies psychopathy. This involves an obfuscation of the need for relationship and a desire to coerce and control others (Meloy, 1992). Dennis's narcissism is on the more extreme end of the spectrum, where the self is taken as the object and the need for others is replaced by a manipulation and use of it. What he tended to demonstrate through his acts of abuse was a complete denial of the need for others.

These disturbing aspects of psychopathy did not form all of Dennis's narrative. His story is also one of loss; at heart, the loss of a mother who could have given Dennis the holding and containment needed for him to develop a protective psychic skin (Bick, 1968). This central loss was compounded by a series of environmental failures resulting in the loss for him of a sense of childhood and, underpinning this, the loss of the notion of a non-disabled self. Just as every parent of a baby with disabilities allows themselves tantalising and agonising fantasies of what their baby would have been like if their brains had not been starved of oxygen, subject to injury or imbalanced by the wrong ratio of chromosomes, forensic disability patients hold an encapsulated fantasy of the kind of life they would have lived were their brains not encumbered by handicap. These tend (particularly but not exclusively when related in group analytic settings) to be conceptualised as a twin phantasy. One member of a forensic group for paedophiles with intellectual disabilities spoke with the group of having swallowed his twin whole, while both were in the womb. I was taken aback by the detail and certainty of his fantasy, while the other group members tended to concur that this had also happened to them. This group phantasy allowed us to think about these incorporated twins as containing all of the men's potentials. While there was some disagreement as to whether eating up the twin had resulted in the dead twin's intelligence being digested, there was no disagreement that the imagined twin's intelligence was high, and that they symbolised for the men a version of a life unlived. In examining these notions of twinship, the men were able to begin to look at the third secret—mortality, and the need to mourn the loss of the intelligent self they could never be.

The inability to mourn is a key diagnostic feature of perversion, and one that connects closely with the difficulties faced by patients with intellectual disabilities in processing death, both in the concrete and the symbolic. Blackman (2003) has written of the myriad ways people with intellectual disabilities are removed from death, ostensibly as a paternalistic way of protecting them from trauma, but in ways that actually serve to re-traumatise them. One patient I worked with many years ago circled the death of her mother in session after session, never quite exorcising her painfully confused feelings of shame, exacerbated by her sibling's refusal to allow her to attend the funeral. "They were scared I'd make a fuss," she said, eventually. "Like I was going to make a mess. Like it was my fault." For her the failure to be part of the rituals of grief prevented true and necessary mourning from taking place. She lived with an agonising and tantalising sense of her mother being half alive and half dead, her own absence from her mother's graveside making it almost impossible for her to place her mother in the grave and move on with her own life.

Dennis's sexual enactments may be understood as communications of his core struggle with the three secrets. At its heart his story is, like that of so many forensic patients, about the unbearable nature of anxiety and loss. My assessment of him clarified his need for these three secrets to be thought about by him and by those around him. Forensic psychotherapy with patients with disabilities is a systemic as well as a psychoanalytic project where the connections between a patient's acts of abuse and their history of exploitation, abuse and neglect have to be formed into a narrative that can be understood not just by the patient, but by those he relies upon for his care. We aim to exist in a state of psychic homeostasis (Freud, 1916–1917) in which we feel our self to be enough to withstand internal anxieties and dangers from outside. Dennis's psychic skin was porous, lacking the integrity to provide him with a sense of protection against the vicissitudes of the world. He had come to need his perversion as a form of pseudo-skin, with any threat to psychic homeostasis (a blow to self-esteem, a humiliation, or a loss) provoking a perverse enactment (Doctor, 2003). An added factor in his psychopathology was his failure to symbolise. Dennis thought concretely at all times, and lacked the capacity to take in any "as if" interpretations. Feeling sad did not evoke in him thoughts such as, "It's *as if* I'm losing everything"—he *was*, in his mind, losing everything, to the point where the normal frustrations and disappointments of everyday life were experienced as annihilatory attacks on his self.

Dennis demonstrates many aspects of the forensic disability patient. His sexual offending was a defence against intimacy, and had been compounded by his struggle to integrate his relationship with disability, sexuality and loss. The aetiology of his enactments was rooted in environmental, relational and traumatogenic factors. Using the concept of the core complex (Glasser, 1979) we can see Dennis's longing for an enmeshed closeness to another, representing a "state of oneness". For him the merger was felt to be permanent, bringing with it a loss of self and the death of him as an individual. The desire for merger became conflated with annihilatory anxiety, with normal, ordinary closeness, and intimacy becoming replaced by all pervading fear. He could oscillate between closeness being seen as annihilating and aloneness being seen as a dismal sentence of lifelong solitary confinement. He had little concept of a safe emotional distance between himself and others. Either the object of desire ejected him alone into the wilderness or was a gag that would suffocate him. He had used sexualised aggression as an agent to provide some semblance of safety. His wish to hurt and humiliate others in sexual ways was his only way of protecting himself from his own pain and humiliation, with sexual aggression becoming a container for his unbearable anxiety.

Armed with this knowledge of the aetiology of Dennis's perversions, how should we expect to treat him? One of our initial responses to a perpetrator with intellectual disabilities is to treat with cruelty or kindness, or with a curious amalgam of the two. Cruelty is more available to us, not just because of our unconscious desire to punish those whose perverse acts remind us of our own buried pockets of perversion, objectification and cruelty, but because we are part of a society that has created structures and containers in which the punishment of the perverse can be easily enacted. It would, of course, be easy to lock Dennis away and, indeed, at the time of assessment, it was hard to see how he could avoid eventually ending up in a prison cell.

Prevalence studies of forensic disability patients in prison are complicated by diagnostic variations and inconsistencies in how the Criminal Justice System assesses and records evidence of disability. International studies have shown a large range, from two per cent to forty per cent, depending on methodological approaches (Jones, 2007). Whatever the figure, one does not need to be in a prison to feel imprisoned. There are a far higher number of forensic disability patients subject to a new form of social imprisonment that is unfettered from considerations of natural justice and human rights. To have an intellectual disability and to be suspected of committing some form of sexual abuse makes you terribly vulnerable to imprisonment without any form of due process. My caseload has included patients who live under a regime of social imprisonment, in which they are escorted everywhere by one, two, or three members of staff. Articles 6 to 11 of the Declaration of Human Rights state that:

6. Everyone has the right to recognition everywhere as a person before the law.
7. All are equal before the law and are entitled without any discrimination to equal protection of the law. All are entitled to equal protection against any discrimination in violation of this Declaration and against any incitement to such discrimination.
8. Everyone has the right to an effective remedy by the competent national tribunals for acts violating the fundamental rights granted him by the constitution or by law.
9. No one shall be subjected to arbitrary arrest, detention or exile.
10. Everyone is entitled in full equality to a fair and public hearing by an independent and impartial tribunal, in the determination of his rights and obligations and of any criminal charge against him.

11. Everyone charged with a penal offence has the right to be presumed innocent until proved guilty according to law in a public trial at which he has had all the guarantees necessary for his defence. No one shall be held guilty of any penal offence on account of any act or omission which did not constitute a penal offence, under national or international law, at the time when it was committed. Nor shall a heavier penalty be imposed than the one that was applicable at the time the penal offence was committed.

In the most shocking but far from rare cases I have worked on, the alleged act of sexual crime has been revealed to have never happened, to have been instead an enactment of sexual confusion or a response to unbearable sexual frustration arising from a life of enforced abstinence. Despite this, and although those accused have undergone no due process, they have no freedom. They are prisoners without trial, alarmingly vulnerable to arbitrary arrest, detention, or exile.

Forensic disability therapy has been born, nurtured and developed against the odds, being a discipline that seeks to work with patients who too many clinicians regard as untreatable on two unalterable counts—their disability and their forensic history. I have used theoretical concepts from both forensic and disability domains to explore the aetiology of abuse perpetrated by patients with intellectual disabilities, and, in doing so, have used the experience of working with "Dennis" to examine the interplay between early object relational ruptures (Glasser, 1979) and the forensic disability patient's ongoing struggles with the "three secrets" (Hollins & Grimer, 1988) of disability, sexuality, and death. I have been forced to conclude that loss, as much as anxiety, lies at the perverse heart of our patients' actions, and a collective failure to recognise this has caused many forensic patients to be on the receiving end of a brutal form of social imprisonment, rather than the treatment they need. The law is notoriously disabled when dealing with people with intellectual disabilities, whether they are victims, perpetrators, or have committed no crime, and struggles to find ways of understanding the patient's perverse actions. I wish now to examine ways in which the narrative of the patient's perverse acts can be understood in a way that is cognisant of the many layers of trauma underpinning the act itself, and which can create a narrative that provides meaning not just to us, but to the forensic disability patient himself.

CHAPTER TWO

Mapping the unknown world: a narrative approach to risk assessment

Risk assessment is an attempt to formulate risk, profile the alleged perpetrator and examine ways in which risk factors can be managed. It is a process made more complex when the patient is acutely disturbed, presenting some form of mental disturbance (Duggan, 1997), and requires a particularly sophisticated formulation when the patient has an intellectual disability. In this chapter I will examine ways in which the risk presented by forensic patients with intellectual disabilities can be analysed and responded to using a narrative approach. A risk assessment represents an opportunity to create a coherent account, one of the defining features of the narrative form (Linde, 1993), and should, I argue, be regarded primarily as a co-authored story, with the assessor, the patient and his support network being seen as "joint authors". I will use anonymised clinical vignettes to explore the notion of risk assessment as an intersubjective process, the result of a clinical interaction between not only assessor and assessed, but also members of what I call the "triangular square". I will examine ways in which the dyadic nature of assessment can be modified to incorporate a more systemic perspective, and will consider the particularly powerful forms of countertransference that are encountered in assessing forensic patients with intellectual disabilities.

Sexual abuse attacks social norms and puts outrage, horror, and confusion into all those who experience or hear about it—apart from the perpetrator himself, who tends to be insulated from these normal responses by tightly constructed defences of minimisation and denial. When we hear about sexual abuse perpetrated by someone with an intellectual disability a heightened sense of confusion tends to be evoked. While it is undoubtedly difficult for a non-abuser to understand why anyone would commit an act of sexual abuse, we struggle even more to comprehend its meaning when disability is involved. Hence the need for a process by which meaning can be made. Without the meaning-making of narrative, perversion is a set of random acts, existing in a split-off vacuum. This may well have been enough for the patient, as the perverse excitement and power evoked by their actions may partially compensate for their lack of meaning. It cannot be enough for us. Without narrative, we are at risk of operating from the same mindless place as the patient, treating offences as split-off actions, separate from the emotional world of the patient. Risk assessment is more than a map with which we can navigate the deeper recesses of our patient's internal world, and more complex than a framework with which levels of risk and danger can be codified. All that happens in the assessment space (including interactions with the triangular square) contributes towards a construction of a narrative that adds meaning to action, which focuses by necessity on areas of perversion and risk, while also teaching us something about the internal landscape of our patients.

Buchanan (1999) delineates approaches to risk assessment as being the actuarial and the clinical—the former quantitative, the latter qualitative, with an inevitable and necessary overlap between the two. The former approach has produced a range of manualised assessment tools both in relation to the general forensic population and those with intellectual disabilities. "Risk containment" (Monahan, 1993) describes the need for a multifaceted systemic response to danger, while Snowden (1997) considers risk assessment (primarily though not exclusively non-sexual) from three perspectives:

i. Risk identification
ii. Frequency and severity
iii. Clinical risk management.

The approach I will describe in this chapter is a largely qualitative process. Just as I have described disability therapy as a deeply intersubjective endeavour (Corbett, 2011), I wish to extend this to the assessment process as well. Risk assessment is not simply an account by one about another. It is created through a clinical interaction, an interpersonal exchange guided as much by unconscious factors as conscious facts. At the heart of the assessment is the dyad: the assessor and the assessed. Every report has a longer list of credits, including not just those who have provided concrete information about the patient's history, but all those whose words, attitudes or silences have subtly shaped the assessor's perceptions. It is important to delineate between these two realms of hard and soft information, with each hard conclusion needing to be evidenced, particularly if the assessment is to be used as part of a legal process, and each soft hypothesis being contextualised in the data from which it has emerged.

A full risk assessment cannot be conducted without the consent of the patient. Where consent is not given, a far more limited analysis of the forensic history may be undertaken, but its results and findings are inevitably weakened by the absence of the protagonist of the forensic narrative. Patients should not be regarded as either having or not having the capacity to consent. From a legal perspective, the presence of an intellectual disability does not mean the patient cannot consent. Given the centrality of consent or its lack thereof in every act of abuse, the patient's understanding of what consent is must be examined from a clinical perspective. To what extent a forensic patient is able to conceptualise consent may help inform us about their capacity to understand the consequences of actions and their ability to consider the right of a subject to say no to something—healthy or perverse—being done to them.

With the patient we are seeking to ascertain how much they understand about the reasons for the assessment, and how they comprehend what the benefits and risks could be. Taking a human rights perspective requires of us an authentic attempt to think with the patient about the benefits for them, rather than for society (although the two may also be seen to be inextricably linked). Society may see a benefit of conducting the assessment as greater safety for potential victims. This may be achieved through, for example, a higher level of supervision and monitoring of the patient. The patient may view this as a risk. Who, after all, would wish to sign up to a process by which their freedom of movement will be restricted? There is at the heart of all risk assessments a paradox of the patient being encouraged to open himself up in the service of a process that could be used "against" him (Van Velson, 2010). Perhaps the most powerful way of addressing this fraught area of benefits versus risk is to talk with the patient about the risk assessment representing their opportunity to tell their story for the first time. While this may hold little weight for those patients who have been through innumerable previous assessments, for others this may be the first time they have voiced their narrative, the first time someone has listened to and witnessed their history.

Risk assessment reports have the power to help ensure the safety of potential victims of sexual abuse who should be regarded as our primary concern. As authors of these reports we also have a responsibility towards the alleged perpetrator, as a forensic label can be branded indelibly upon someone for years, colouring and shaping attitudes towards them and compromising their access to normal aspects of everyday life. There is a particular risk of over documenting risk so that the label is tattooed upon the patient forever. To ensure the forensic assessment process is, as far as possible, an objective one requires careful thought about baseline terminology. Most assessments have a particular grammar and vocabulary, with "high" "medium" and "low" risk labels used to provide clarity as to the potential level of danger posed by patients. There is a risk of each of these labels being interpreted in an overly subjective way—a risk exacerbated if there is no global agreement on their various meanings. Without a baseline we are tremendously vulnerable to anxiety informing our findings. The patient is in danger of being split off as bad, "high risk", allowing the organisation, and the clinicians within it, some relief from their complex feelings of anxiety and responsibility. Antebi (2003) describes the dangers implicit in assuming the mantle of crime prevention officer by which "the hope we should bring to each clinical situation is lost and that will inevitably be experienced by the patient. The consequence of this is an *increase* in dangerousness" (p. 12).

In formulating risk, it is helpful to delineate between the following levels of risk.

Low:	It is improbable that the patient will act out sexually.
Medium:	It is possible the patient will act out sexually.
High:	It is probable the patient will act out sexually.
Very High:	It is improbable the patient will not act out sexually.

In order to reach sound conclusions as to a patient's level of risk, a set of processes need to be carried out:

i. Pre-referral interaction instigated by the patient's support network ascertaining the suitability of the assessor for conducting the assessment
ii. Consent negotiations covering consent for engagement in the assessment
iii. Collation of psychological, educational, social and health reports
iv. Bio psychosocial consultation involving representatives of the patient's support team, and family, where appropriate
v. Forensic interviews with the patient
vi. Collation of forensic report
vii. Meeting with support team to discuss findings and implementation plan.

Indicators as to the forensic patient's narrative tend to be glimpsed in the process of how he is referred to risk assessment. Anxiety underpins most forensic referrals, often serving to dampen the capacity to think. Referrals are often made for treatment rather than assessment, with the referrers acting on a sense of extreme urgency despite there having been, in many cases, years of inertia and inaction preceding the point of referral. Our starting question has then to be: Why now? What factors are in place now to make this referral possible, and what has happened to make inertia untenable? Has the patient projected his anxieties into the team, relieving him of the need to deal with them? Why do the team seem to want the patient to be treated without working out what needs to be treated? The answers to these questions begin our vari-focal assessment as they alert us to the psychodynamics of the patient's external world. To adapt the notion of there being no such thing as "just a baby" (Winnicott, 1964), there is no such thing as *just* a forensic disability patient. There is always a forensic disability patient in relation to his support network. With some patients this will be their family; with others it will be the team in the group home where they live, or the daycentre where they spend most of their time. Whichever, the risk assessment will need to build a bridge to them, prior to the assessment beginning. This bridge will allow the transmission of important information such as, for example, the facts and quality of the patient's childhood, the nature of their current attachments and the way in which they deal with anxiety.

The bridge should also allow something equally important to be learnt: how does the patient make people feel? Does the family feel disabled by him? Does he evoke parental shame? Is he loved? Are there significant differences within the team in terms of how they feel about him? With the team, as with the family, we may be able to learn something important about the patient's internal world through noticing how much splitting occurs around them. We are all vulnerable to splitting between the good and bad as part of the human struggle to navigate our way from the paranoid-schizoid states of early infanthood towards a more nuanced view of our internal and external worlds as being a complex but manageable blend of the desired and the feared (Klein, 1946). To be able to hold an ambivalent sense of ourselves and the world around us is a necessary developmental task. The forensic patient tends not to be able to tolerate or withstand ambivalence, reverting to a primitive and highly split state where the gulf between the good and the bad cannot be symbolised in a healthy way, leading to concrete and sometimes aggressive enactments. Vulnerability to this form of extreme splitting is not the sole domain of the forensic patient; it can be projected into all aspects of their support network.

This split between good and bad is all too easily evacuated into those surrounding the patient, resulting in a profound form of forensic splitting within and between teams. The patient's perverse desire to destroy and be destroyed finds a home in settings where the balance between overly rigid thinking and loose inconsistency is hard to maintain. Just as viruses flourish in immunodeficient bodies, forensic splitting is most alive in settings prone to poor communication, in which anxiety is uncontained and where fear tends to be the default emotional setting. Hopper's fourth basic assumption (2003a, 2003b), by which teams, groups and organisations defend against the trauma they work with through an inauthentic "group think" or massification, is particularly apposite in the field of forensic disability therapy. What cannot be avoided is the inevitability of patients projecting their psychopathology into teams. What can be developed is a more robust container for such attacks. Any assessment of risk must be vari-focal, with a capacity to focus on both the external as well as the internal world of the forensic patient.

Identifying the abused within the abuser is a necessary component of forensic psychotherapy and assessment, as it provides a methodological framework for understanding the aetiology of sexual crime. By abuse, I am not just considering experiences of sexual abuse, but encompassing equally traumatising experiences of severe neglect and deprivation. Identifying the abusing parts of a patient is also essential—we need to be clear about what our patients have done and what they are capable of doing. Seeing just one aspect, be it the abused or the abuser, threatens to blind us to the complexity of our patient's psychopathology, and either blunts our analytic capacity by forcing us to attune solely to the victim within the victimiser, or sharpens us to the point where we can only interact with our patients through cruelty and denigration.

To conduct a forensic assessment with a patient with intellectual disabilities necessitates a parallel assessment of the milieu in which they live, and an evaluation of the forms of splitting processes that may therein exist. Noticing such processes provides insight into what the patient projects into those around him, and what is projected back into him. It is also a component of the assessment process by which we are assessing the capacity of the patient's carers to support the patient throughout the assessment process. Where the team and/or family is too split, or too massified, it is likely that they may collapse under the strain of the patient's assessment (teams may enact their ambivalence through sabotaging the assessment by causing the patient to always be late or overmedicated for sessions, or may consistently "forget" the appointments). In such cases an organisational and/or family consultancy may be required to get the matrix to a healthier position. In some cases the pre-assessment stage reveals a scapegoating process by which the patient is carrying a set of symptoms on behalf of the matrix. The supposed index offence may have been acted out of confusion about boundaries or the result of a lack of education, devoid of an intent to abuse. It may be the visible leaking of a family dynamic suffused with blurred and broken sexual boundaries. It may be the signifier of a residential setting in which all sexual boundaries held by staff and patients have been merged. In such cases the treatment spotlight is turned upon the family or the residential setting. They hold the mantle of forensic patient. Just as anxiety lies at the heart of the forensic enactment, institutions are vulnerable to defending against the anxiety of their staff and require particularly sensitive clinical interventions to enable them to look at and deal with these anxieties (Menzies Lyth, 1988).

Welldon (1996a) links the forensic patient's fears of intimacy in a one-to-one situation with their need to engage in a process of triangulation in which they are not just engaged with their therapist, they also form a strong attachment to the setting in which the therapist works. Scheffer (1996) sees this as the symbolic representation of the original mother–father–child relationship, providing, in a metaphysical sense, the potential for the optimal development of a "holding environment" (Winnicott, 1965a). What these, and others (Evans, Carlyle & Dolan, 1996), mean when they refer to the triangular involvement of a third party in forensic psychotherapy is the inclusion of society in the treatment of offenders. As we have seen, with patients with intellectual disabilities there is a fourth party made up of the patient's care network. Sometimes this involves family members, sometimes members of staff charged with supporting the patient within their residential setting. Thus we are working with a matrix that has echoes of the square triangular number in mathematics, where a number is both a triangular number and a perfect square. The dyad of the patient and therapist is connected to and with the setting in which the therapy is conducted, the setting in which the patient is cared for, and, surrounding the matrix, the society in which the patient and the therapist exist. All assessment of forensic patients with intellectual disabilities exists therefore in a triangular square.

Once the triangular square has been constructed, the next stage is the gathering of history about the patient and their alleged abuses. Information such as educational, social and family history, records of previous allegations, and previous psychological assessments are valuable metanarratives with which to contextualise the patient. Attention should be paid to the role of diagnosis. The certainty with which previous assessors have described the patient's level of disability or the presence of mental health diagnoses can blind us to the subjectivity of diagnosis. It is not unusual for one patient to be seen as having a moderate intellectual disability by one clinician, and a severe disability by another. A tentative wondering in a case conference by a trainee psychiatrist as to the possibility of a personality disorder may be dutifully minuted, to be read as an unquestioned psychiatric diagnosis a decade later. All documentation about the forensic patient should be subject to its own forensic analysis.

The risk assessment of a forensic disability patient should take place in as neutral a setting as possible, free from associations with the patient's everyday life. The more severe the patient's disability is the more use they may need to make of creative tools, such as dolls, sand trays, and art materials. Some patients may ask that their carer is with them throughout the assessment process. Ideally, this should be restricted to the beginning of the process, in recognition of the patient's levels of anxiety and the risk of the presence of a carer throughout the whole assessment diluting the objectivity and neutrality of the process.

The tendency for disability services to adopt an overly insular attitude is particularly marked in relation to risk assessment. The anxiety that drives so many interactions with forensic issues tends to drive many settings to seek to deal with forensic issues "in house". This is undoubtedly connected to the shame services can feel when abuse happens within their walls—a shame that cathects with the disability transference (see Chapter Five) by which the ability to process thought is affected and distorted by the relationship with disability itself. Too often services suffer a breakdown in thinking and minimise the importance of acts of sexual perversion by seeking to assess risk themselves. While this does not render the entire process untenable, it removes objectivity and neutrality from the process, reducing the possibility of a full narrative being uncovered. Where possible the form of risk assessment described here should be undertaken by a clinician outside the organisation, free from its internal dynamics.

* * *

"Daniel", thirty-two, enters the consulting room like a brick smashing through a window. The room races from silence to noise in the time it takes him to slam the door behind him. Although I have been briefed about his manic, loud, ferocious state, I still feel that something has smashed into me. He is a tall, ungainly man, dressed in a suit two sizes too small for him. His face is flushed and he is breathless, as if he has run all the way here. I start to introduce myself, but he does not want to hear who I am, he only wants to let me know all about his key worker, Josh.

"Josh came with me," he says. "He didn't have to but he wanted to. I can come on my own. He's nice to me. Do you know him? He says he knows you. He says you're nice. He's nice too. I don't have to come if I don't want to. Stopped in cafe round the corner. I had coffee. Two sugars. Lots of milk. Not too hot. Josh drinks tea. No sugar. Little bit of milk. Nice and hot, thank you very much!"

He talks for another five minutes or so, sometimes sitting down opposite me but more often leaping up and scouring the room for clues as to what it is for. He picks up dolls, runs his fingers through the sand tray and looks through the blinds at the building opposite. I find myself feeling breathless, as if his manic, accelerated way of being has already been deposited inside me. He pauses for breath, and I say "How good to meet you. You've got so much to tell me. How are we going to fit it all in? We've got today, and then we've got eleven more sessions after that and you're already making sure you cram it all in before it ends. Let me say something about who I am."

He sits down briefly, but then leaps up again, and continues his monologue, telling me more about Josh's likes and dislikes, what shifts he has worked this week, when his next holiday is coming up, and what colour car he drives. Eventually there is another tiny pause, and I leap in, wanting to take the opportunity before it vanishes. "My name's Alan," I say. He starts to talk again, but I continue. "I'm wondering if you're really worried about finding out who I am, or about letting me know who you are. We could be here until ten to three without me knowing anything about you and you knowing nothing about me. I think that would be awful. It would be really terrible if your worries stopped us from properly meeting each other." He slows down somewhat, giving me the chance to ask him why he thinks he is here. "Josh said," he replies, inevitably. "I wonder if you think I will be so much more interested in Josh than I will be in you," I say. He looks blank for a moment, and I reflect that I am probably wrong. "Or maybe you're scared I *will* be interested in you—maybe you don't want me to think about you, and why you're here." Some of his manic bravado fades away, and he sits still for the first time.

He does, in fact, look more humiliated than frightened, but I choose to take up the notion of fear, judging humiliation to be a concept that may be too dense for him to be able to digest at this point in the assessment. I explain that many people who come here are frightened—often because they've done frightening things and are scared of getting into trouble. I let him know that I think it would be good if he could stay in the room even when he gets scared so that we can talk about his fears. I also say that if the fears get too much, or if any feelings get too much, he can leave the room." "See Josh?" he says, wistfully. I nod. "Yes, if things feel too bad, you could see Josh."

Daniel has been referred because of a long history of sexually assaulting boys and girls. His offences mirror his presence in the consulting room. He crashes into the child's space, not allowing them to breathe, to scream or to run away. He is quick in all he does. He can escape the gaze of his one-to-one worker in the time it takes for the worker to check their phone for messages. He can identify the child he wishes to abuse within seconds, seeming to have a perverse form of radar with which he picks up the child whose internal landscape most closely resembles his own—alone, unsupported, easy to lose. His offending is as violent as it is quick, and his skill in ensuring children are muted by their terror of him mean his forensic history has remained under cover for many years.

By the end of the second session I think that Daniel understands what the assessment is for, and knows he can withdraw from it if it feels as if it is destroying his carefully constructed defences. The third session starts with him telling me as much as he can remember about his childhood. He is the middle of three children, all of whom have some form of developmental disorder. His parents are still alive, though now elderly and see him rarely. When I try to explore any thoughts or feelings about them, he shuts down, or more often lets me know that Josh is his key worker now—he is good, he is friendly. He is most alive when talking about Josh, and I start to ask about the other people in the home where he lives, about whom he has been silent. "They're lots of stupid," he says, with a sigh. "Not clever like me. Don't like them." This confirms what his team have told me: that he is isolated and alone within the home, seeming to regard his fellow residents with disdain and saving all his attention and affection for members of staff. I note, but do not say, how much Daniel may need to evacuate his loathing of his disability into others so he can maintain a protective fiction that he is more like his carers than his peers.

Daniel's vocabulary is limited, and he tends to default to bland, inoffensive words with which to describe the quality of his relationships. "Mum and dad were nice," "my brothers are good," "my room is ok." There is no life or vitality in his language, and I start to worry away at this with him. "Mum and dad were nice," I echo, adding "but everyone seems nice. You're allowed to tell me when people or things aren't nice." This is an especially important nudge to give any forensic patient with disabilities, as they are likely to conform to Bybee and Zigler's (1999) theory of outer directedness, whereby people with intellectual disabilities are prone to be overly compliant, avoiding any expressions of unhappiness or non conformity that might cause others to be unhappy. The handicapped smile (Sinason, 1986) is not just a defence against trauma, it is also a way of eliciting a smile rather than a sneer in return.

I ask Daniel to tell me what life was like when he was little. He looks blank, little thought showing in his features, and eventually replies, "Nice. It was nice." Something more authentic emerges when he brings his photograph album into the session. We look at this together, and I am struck by his partial absence from most of the pictures. He was always on the move, a blurry jumble of colours dashing from the lens, or held firmly by his father—the tense faces on both father and son betraying a pre-picture drama to ensure he didn't escape from the clutches of the camera. The pictures also seem to me to show a disabled family. Both parents share a similar look of stupefaction that suggests a couple united by disability who had somehow managed to keep their family afloat and outside the support of social services. This is a thought that I do voice to Daniel—"Mum and dad look like they might have had disabilities too." Daniel looks shocked, and tells me that "Mum was sometimes stupid, but dad wasn't ... Dad was in charge ... Dad hit anyone who did anything stupid." We spend some time on these photographs which act as a prompt to me to ask whether what I think I am seeing on people's expressions matches what Daniel remembers. A narrative of domestic violence emerges, with Daniel gradually becoming more able to describe a childhood of terror in which the father bound his family together through acts of severe and unpredictable sadism.

This is the first time Daniel has talked about his father in this way, and his tightly held defences of stoic niceness erode. He allows himself to cry, before quickly pulling himself together and saying "Crying's stupid. Crying doesn't make it better." I hear his father's cruel tone in Daniel's voice, and I understand something more about how he has internalised his father's disdain for stupidity, weakness, and vulnerability.

When we talk about the children who have alleged he has abused them, Daniel gives voice to his father once more: "They're stupid. Making it up. Not nice." I remind him that this is his chance to tell his side of the story: "Children keep saying you've hurt them—let's think about the last time this happened."

Daniel describes a social worker coming to his home to tell him a little girl had said he had hurt her. He talks about his anger towards the "stupid girl" and I ask him to tell me more about how stupid she was. The split between Daniel's disabled and non-disabled parts becomes painfully clear. He draws a verbal picture of this girl as a manipulative, dishonest monster, while letting thoughts about her vulnerability, the sad look in her eyes, and how she reminded him of his younger self leak out. Over the course of three further sessions he talks more about one of the days on which he abused this girl. He talks about waking up feeling bad, not knowing what to do with this sense of "badness". He oscillates between a sense of sorrow for himself, and waves of anger towards this girl who, in his mind, forced herself to be abused by him. In his final session he appears deflated, and desperately sad about the narrative that has emerged between us. He shows some anxiety about what happens next: what will I write in my report and who will see it? Finally he simply refuses to leave the consulting room when the time is up. He is unable to say he is attached to me, describing instead his sadness at leaving the "nice room". Eventually, with much coaxing from Josh, he departs.

The chaos of Daniel's internal world is enacted through boundary breaking of the most perverse kind. Risk assessment is, in effect, a study of boundaries, an analysis of how and why they are broken, and an attempt to hypothesise ways of repairing them. No surprise, then, that I conduct this assessment using solid, firm boundaries of time and space, and that Daniel ends by seeking to break them. The "structuring of time" (Cox, 1992, p. 338) is of vital importance in creating the framework of any assessment. The temptation to loosen one's time boundaries with patients with intellectual disabilities stems from what Symington (1992) described as a countertransference response of disdain and hatred. The lack of value given to time reflects the lack of value accorded to those with disabilities, particularly those who are thought to have committed acts of abuse. Welldon (2011) requires clinicians to "always see the patient at the time agreed for the appointment, neither earlier nor later: earlier will be felt as seduction; later as a sense of neglect, repeating the experience of "nobody caring" (p. 160). Although Welldon is speaking here directly about psychotherapy sessions and, in fact, advises that diagnostic meetings should take place at irregular intervals to avoid the intensity of the emergence of the transference, I place equal importance on the time boundary across both disciplines. Forensic disability patients are too vulnerable to embedded anxieties about themselves and their victims not mattering to be able to withstand any suggestion that this is the case through how little we seem to care about their time.

A forensic assessment involving a patient with intellectual disabilities also tends to require more time than non-disability assessments. Daniel's assessment required twelve one-hour meetings, which tends to be the optimum duration in this field. The more disabled the patient the more sessions will be required, and vice versa. This allows for the following six key areas to be examined:

i. Narrative: the patient's story (*"Who are you?"*)
ii. Cognitive: the cognitive processes used in the formation of narrative and relationship, and how a disability impinges upon this (*"What do you understand this assessment to be about?"*)
iii. Affective: the emotional world of the patient (*"How do you feel about being here?"*)
iv. Communicative: how the patient understands and relates to the world (*"How best can we understand each other?"*)
v. Relational: how the patient relates to the assessor (*"Do you know who and what I am?"*)
vi. Forensic: the patient's sexual history—both consensual and non consensual (*"You're here because people are worried. What are they worried about, and does it worry you too?"*)

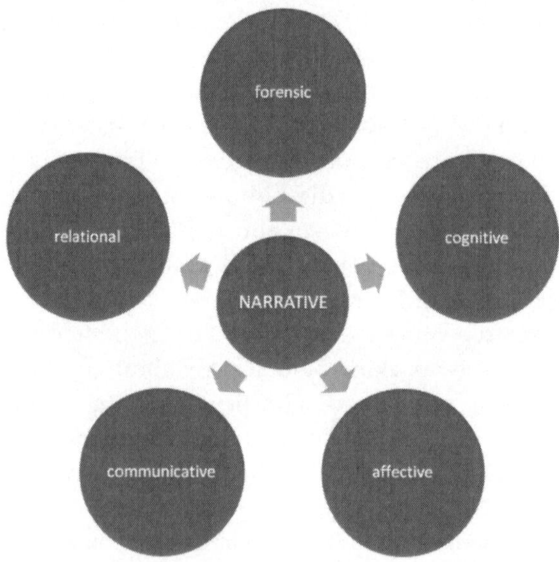

Figure 1. Risk assessment domains.

A key aspect of Daniel's narrative is the presence of humiliation. Gilligan's (1997) studies into violence suggest it is preceded by a pervasive feeling of humiliation, provoking intense feelings of shame that the forensic patient struggles to contain. My decision not to alert Daniel to his feelings of humiliation within the assessment (choosing instead to focus on his feelings of fear) underscore the need for care when choosing what can be interpreted, and what should be left to the work of psychotherapy. By aiming my lens on fear rather than humiliation I was forming a judgment about the nature of Daniel's defences, and how unprepared he may have been to have them dismantled within an investigative rather than a therapeutic process.

I make similar decisions about whether to voice my hypotheses about Daniel's valency for projective identification (his tendency to evacuate his hatred about his own disability into those around him). My caution stemmed from an uncertainty about his capacity to introject interpretations in helpful ways, particularly in the short-term context of the assessment. I do not wish to deconstruct his defences without having time to reconstruct them, or offer some healthier alternatives.

The most purely qualitative research tool lies within the relationship between assessed and assessor. While the patient's unconscious landscape is subject to the most attention, this should not cause the unconscious of the assessor to be neglected. The countertransference is a mixture between a lens and a barometer—magnifying both how feelings are thought about and felt; how they appear and what temperature they reach. Sitting in a room with a patient with an intellectual disability tends to evoke the disability transference (Corbett, 2009) in which one's capacity to think and to communicate may be disabled through a projective evacuation of non-thinking and anti-communication from the patient (see Chapter Five). All that occurs within the consulting room is a communication, the reading of encoded messages between the unconscious of the assessed and the unconscious of the assessor. The more somatic the communication the less connected the patient may be of its meaning of the communication. Anxiety is the driving force behind much psychopathology, but the forensic patient may struggle to recognise or acknowledge its presence. Its presence in the consulting room may be evident only to the therapist. The patient avoids contact with these troublesome feelings through the use of manic defences. The bodily countertransference (Orbach, 2003) is as vital a part of the assessment process as the cognitive. There were points during sessions with Daniel when I found myself suffused with bodily sensations of numbness; other times when I found myself disturbed by unwelcome feelings of sexual arousal that seemed to be able to coexist with cognitive thoughts of non arousal and revulsion. A truly in-depth assessment invites the patient's narrative to be communicated on more than one level, and projected into more than one domain. If the narrative cannot be put into words it may need to be put into the body, and it follows that when the narrative is about sex and part-object relating, we may find our bodies filled up with a visceral, toxic, and perverse sexual countertransference. This then needs to be processed outside of the session, requiring a supervisory stance that is multi-dimensional and that can think of the body as being as potent an assessment tool as the mind.

This may also be the place to think about how we clothe the body we assess with. I have been disturbed in my supervisory practice by a lack of thought given to the impact of our bodies and their clothing upon our patients. An overly casual way of dressing may stem from an egalitarian wish to avoid appearing too powerful within the asymmetrical power dynamic of the clinical dyad. On a less conscious level it may link more to Symington's (1992) notion of the ease with which our hatred of and contempt towards our disabled patients gets transmitted through not caring enough about how we dress with them. It may also be a generous attempt to overcompensate for our shame about having the means to dress ourselves how we want—something that is often denied to people with intellectual disabilities. Whatever the aetiology, we need to avoid dress that shows too much skin, something the forensic patient may simply be unable to deal with. This is a genderless point, as provocative male clothing is as difficult for the forensic patient to deal with as provocative female clothing. Working with forensic patients with intellectual disabilities requires sensitivity to how hard they may find it to regulate desire. Most patients are being assessed because of a propensity to act rather than think, and they deserve and need protection from any further attacks on the capacity to reflect in the assessment space.

My openness to allowing Daniel to bring his photographs into the session was deliberate. It was not just that photographs can be an invaluable therapeutic as well as an investigative clinical tool (Berman, 1993); forensic patients with intellectual disabilities require higher levels of facilitation in forming their narrative than patients without. This may involve the use of dolls, art materials, sand trays, or music.

One of the most powerful narratives I have worked with was that of a fourteen-year-old boy, referred to the clinic in which I worked because of a series of seemingly unprovoked sadistic sexual attacks on younger children in his school. His intellectual disability was severe, and he had few words with which to form a narrative. His receptive skills were enough for him to understand me, as long as I kept my language at the level of a six-year-old. He said little, and we spent many sessions engaged in play. It was mostly one-sided play, for he found it difficult to think of me as really existing in his world. I tried to interpret his play as best I could, with little indication that anything I said was of value to him, or was actually being taken in at all. I found myself feeling some curiosity in him, but it was often diluted by a sense of weariness, a fear that there would be no real exchange from him to me, and that we could both conclude the risk assessment without any narrative sense of why he had done what he had.

It was only when he began to play with a wooden doll's house, and the dolls within it, that a real narrative emerged. He was interested in the look of the house, and seemed to hear me when I said that some children liked to use the house to show me something about the kind of house they grew up in. This acted as a kind of detonator, as he suddenly began to shake the house violently, the dolls inside falling out of the windows and the furniture clanking around, creating a volley of machine gun-like noise. He continued this until the end of the session, and into the next. It emerged that his childhood had been dominated by a violent stepfather, who had used violence to subdue this boy into receiving his sexual advances. The boy, however, never put this into words, and could only communicate it through using auxiliary means. He continued the narrative he had begun in his assessment in his subsequent therapy, eventually using the dolls to show and explore what it had felt like to be like a powerless, terrified ragdoll being thrown around the world by this sadistic adult.

It is moments such as this point of detonation that form the catalyst for the emergence of narrative, particularly, but not exclusively, with patients with more severe disabilities. In this particular case there was little indication that this might happen, with the narrative only arising from a fairly lengthy period of non-directive play. I had, in fact, found myself giving up on the idea of narrative at this point, as I doubted this boy would ever be able to shed light on his seemingly random acts of sexual aggression. So his narrative came to life at a point of giving up—a playing out, perhaps, of a parent giving up on him—his explosions of sexual acting out becoming his only real way of becoming fully alive.

Writing a risk assessment narrative requires a return to the six domains mentioned earlier: narrative, cognitive, affective, communicative, relational and forensic. "Narrative" will form the main overarching thread of the assessment report, documenting as it does the patient's life in chronological form. The narrative domain begins pre-birth. Knowing as we do the powerful influence upon psychopathology of intergenerational abuse, we need to have been interested in the story of previous generations, both from the perspective of our patient and those around him. Attention also needs to be given to the circumstances of the patient's birth. How yearned for were they? How much grief was felt when their disability became apparent? Was the child given "good enough" (Winnicott, 1965b) love, or responded to with rage, disappointment, and hatred? Was it responded to with, in Kleinian terms, the paranoid-schizoid position (a psychic catastrophe that has to be either denied or hated) or the depressive position (where the loss of the longed for, non-disabled baby can be tempered by a sense of authentic hope and love)? A psychosocial perspective should also be given within this narrative, looking at the economic status of the family, an important component of the narrative that will have had an impact upon the family's capacity to survive the detonated bomb that disability can represent. Disability is not just an intrapsychic or interpersonal phenomenon. It touches on painfully real external realities, with most families finding themselves having to battle an increasingly impoverished benefits system to get basic support needs met.

The cognitive narrative domain refers to the role and function of intelligence in the patient's presentation. Here quantitative data may be used as long as it is contextualised alongside qualitative findings. Daniel's IQ was measured as being 52, which defined him as being at the less able end of the spectrum of mild intellectual disability. However, the course of the assessment revealed pockets of higher intelligence, coexisting with pockets of more profound disability—mostly created or impacted by trauma. In assessing this area, it was important to be attuned to the countertransference, noticing those moments where the impact of the disability transference was particularly acute—moments that tended to correlate to parts of the narrative that touched on affects such as shame, humiliation, and anger. The aim of the cognitive narrative is not just to place a patient somewhere on the spectrum of disability; it is an opportunity to think about the impact of disability upon the patient and those around him. Attention should be paid to the patient's primary handicap and their secondary handicap—which has emerged as an exaggeration of the primary disability as a defence mechanism to protect against traumatic memories and feelings (Sinason, 1986). Although Sinason uses the term "opportunistic" in relation to the secondary handicap, she is still describing a predominantly unconscious process. I would like to suggest the term "expedient disability" to describe the forensic patient's *conscious* exaggeration of a primary deficit. This may be used to groom victims (appearing child-like in order to play with children or suggesting guilelessness while manoeuvring an adult into a victimised position) or to avoid responsibility for actions (to appear too "stupid" to have carried out acts of exploitation and abuse). This concept will be examined in more depth in Chapter Nine.

The affective narrative domain refers to the receipt and expression of emotions on the part of the patient. Attention should have been paid to those feelings captured within the countertransference: has the patient made one feel frightened, sad, numb, aroused, stupid, or objectified? In looking at the triangular square, what feelings about the patient were carried there, and how split were they? What kind of emotional vocabulary does the patient possess—particularly in relation to their alleged victims? Does this suggest a capacity for empathy or a more worrying incapacity to consider or place importance on the emotions of another? With patients who are autistic or have pockets of autistic functioning (and, in fact, other patients as well), this narrative domain will be the one in which to comment on the extent to which the patient has a theory of mind: the ability to consider that someone else has a mind that is different from one's own. The degree of empathy we can excavate within the assessment bears upon both the level of risk we judge to be in place, and the amount of therapeutic work to be done.

The communicative narrative domain covers the non-verbal as well as the verbal. This requires of us an attention to somatic responses, the way in which the patient's narrative is conveyed by and through their body—often more than through their words. Attention should be paid to the forms and qualities of silences—whether they're evidence of internal thought, defensive shutting down, or an indicator of questions being digested and made sense of. Daniel often laughed within his assessment sessions, and some laughter evoked a countertransference response in me of discomfort, as if some laughter was non-defensive, a healthy way of releasing tension or responding to something genuinely funny, while other laughter served as a defence against something too painful, too troubling to let in.

In working on the relational narrative domain, we are looking at transference issues, among other things. What kind of relationship, if any, emerged between assessor and assessed? How much concern was evoked in each about the other? What kind of figure did the assessor seem to resemble for the patient? In examining the ease or unease of the relationship, we are examining the patient's capacity to form a positive attachment as well as their ability to relate to another as a person rather than as a sexualised object. It is in this domain that we need to draw on the findings from the triangular square in order to gain a 360-degree perspective on the variety of relationship dynamics evoked by the patient. Key to this will be an examination of the kind of relationship formed between the patient and his victims. This may be gleaned from reading through witness statements or victim impact reports, or from directly interviewing the victims themselves. It should also be based in part on the ways in which the patient describes these relationships—how much congruent feeling is communicated, how much concern there is for the victim, as compared to how much responsibility is projected into them for the acts of abuse.

The forensic narrative domain covers the details of the alleged acts of abuse, as well as a wider analysis of the patient's sense of sexual identity. By the end of the assessment we should have formed a picture of how the patient relates to himself as a sexual being. This is far more than just a comment on the patient's view of their sexual orientation. We should also be interested in whether the patient has an overly pathologised view of sexuality. This is often magnified for forensic patients with disabilities by a distorted sense of the primal act. Wolfensberger (1987) describes an unconscious view of sex as being a "deathmaking activity", something which has resulted in something disabled and, by definition, something inherently damaged. This intrapsychic phenomenon is magnified by the extra psychic, societal view of the disabled person as embodying something that has to be disdained, hated, and feared, something intra and extra-psychic forces combine to view as the result of intercourse gone wrong. We are also examining the role of fantasy within the forensic domain. Violent or sexual fantasies can be understood as precursors to acts of sexual violence, while also telling us something about the patient's sense of self—a self so diminished it can only feel truly alive when gaining power through making others powerless.

A variety of narratives tend to emerge through the construction of the forensic narrative. A risk assessment can give voice to the narrative of the patient as abused as well as abuser, and it is important that neither narrative is diminished by the other. By this I am warning again of the dangers of splitting, of the narrative of the patient as abused being minimised as a form of justification for their narrative as abuser. While some patients may well need to consciously use their experiences of neglect, deprivation, or abuse to garner sympathy and deflect from the impact of their abusive actions, we need to also be attuned to a different narrative that can use these narrative strands to contextualise their forensic enactments. It should be remembered that these six forensic narrative domains are rarely linear and never separate. We may be discovering what the victim means to the abuser, and, in doing so, we may also be discovering whether the abuser's narcissism is so malign that they can only regard others as objects. We are then working in a number of narrative domains: the relational, the affective, and the forensic.

A risk assessment is followed by the implementation of clinical recommendations which then require regular review to judge their efficacy, and their impact upon the level of risk presented by the patient. Risk is a dynamic phenomenon impacted by dynamic variables. The introduction of psychotherapy to a patient following forensic assessment may cause risk to change dramatically—sometimes, in the early stages of treatment, for the worse rather than for the better. As defences are analysed and lowered, alongside a patient beginning to form a more coherent narrative of their life, hitherto repressed memories, emotions, and thoughts may bubble to the surface. The psychic awakening caused by the start of clinical treatment is therefore something of a poisoned chalice. To take just one aspect of treatment, Sinason's secondary handicap (Sinason, 1986) may well be addressed through the course of treatment, whereby a patient may begin to be relieved of the need to maintain a defensive stupidity with which to numb the pain of cumulative trauma. While this is a clinically positive development, it may result in a rather cleverer perpetrator than was initially seen within the assessment, and an angrier one too.

There have to be comparative factors at play in every forensic assessment; judgements about risk are dependent on a wide range of variable factors, requiring of us an openness to considering the impact of systemic and psychological changes in our patients' lives. Levels of risk fluctuate over time. Our first set of findings must be based on what the risk currently is, and what it will continue to be should no changes be made. If the risk is not low, we must then consider what changes need to be in place to reduce it over time.

Let's look again at the definitions of risk outlined at the start of this chapter:

Low:	It is improbable that the patient will act out sexually.
Medium:	It is possible the patient will act out sexually.
High:	It is probable the patient will act out sexually.
Very High:	It is improbable the patient won't act out sexually.

We can then begin to formulate the kind of recommendations we wish to make in our assessment report, with the level of intervention needed rising incrementally with the level of risk identified. While a low risk may have been identified within the patient, the assessment may have identified that the real forensic problem actually lies within the team. Where there is, for example, a team that has been revealed to be worryingly split, with the patient acting as a mix of scapegoat and container for the team's disavowed confusion, anxiety, and rage, there is a clear need for the team's narrative to be worked with. This may happen through ongoing consultation with them, or through creating supervisory spaces in which these anxious projections can be gradually dismantled and worked through.

As the aetiology of sexual perversion is usually multi-causal, it follows that there is rarely one solution that will reduce the patient's risk. In most cases we need to consider a combination of interventions, such as individual and/or group psychotherapy, psycho-education, family intervention, and supervision and monitoring for higher risk patients. In order to monitor the impact of these recommendations, the formulation of a forensic assessment requires the coming together of a risk management team tasked with continuing the ongoing process of risk evaluation. The membership of this group should include key members of the patient's support team, such as social workers, residential support workers, probation officers, and psychologists. The inclusion of the psychotherapist working with the patient raises a complex question about how far the boundaries of psychotherapy need to be adhered to when working with forensic patients. Hook (2001) advocates psychotherapeutic involvement in case conferences, case reviews, and clinical team meetings to allow the formation of a working relationship that mitigates against the holding of distorted and prejudicial views by different professionals—the clinician as advocate as well as therapist. McGauley and Humphrey (2003) highlight the need for the therapist to maintain an appropriate balance between informing the team of risk factors that may emerge through the clinical work and ensuring an adequate level of confidentiality in the therapeutic process. The forensic disability therapist is often forced to straddle two worlds: attending to their patient who needs, of course, to know that no detail of the content of their therapy can leak outside the consulting room, while being cognisant of the anxieties of the members of the triangular square, and their desperate need to know how the patient is doing in their therapy. To protect the disability therapist from being torn apart by the splitting processes that underpin every forensic case, care should be taken to identify a forensic risk manager who can help protect the boundaries of the therapeutic work while allowing the support teams and families to be alive to changes in levels of risk and danger.

* * *

The core of any assessment is the sexually aggressive act. Our role as clinicians is to promote thinking about the unconscious meaning of the act—both in the patient and in those around him. While the association of crime with unconscious guilt and shame is hardly new in the field of psychoanalysis (Freud, 1916d) and has become the bedrock of contemporary forensic psychotherapy, the disability field, with significant exceptions, continues to view the forensic actions of patients with intellectual disabilities as a largely behavioural phenomenon (Lindsay, 2002; Talbot & Langdon, 2006; MacKinlay & Langdon, 2009). If the provision of psychotherapy to patients with intellectual disabilities is a subversive challenge to the behavioural status quo (Corbett, 2014) a psychoanalytically informed analysis of the aetiology of sexual perversion is a similarly radical act. The meaning of the sexual enactment must be central to any risk assessment, as without it we are merely placing bandages on a deepening wound. Throughout the assessment we must keep alive the notion of the sexual act as a metaphor, the symptom of a pervasive disease. The assessment is an experiment in time travel, as most analyses are; looking to the past (what early and later trauma caused a deviation from the path of normal sexual development), the present (what recent trauma has caused the patient's defences to slip or break) and the future (what does the patient need in order to both process the original trauma and manage the current attacks on their defences).

I have used narrative as a metaphor with which to consider the function of a risk assessment. I suggest that, as with forensic psychotherapy, I am considering risk assessment as a narrative with shared authorship, a co-creation between patient and assessor, aided by engagement with and input from the "triangular square". It is important to conclude with a reminder that risk assessment may never be a full narrative. Just as it can be argued that no psychoanalysis can be deemed to be complete, all risk assessments will have a lacuna. We may strive to uncover the aetiology of a patient's perverse acts, or excavate those of their object relations that have contributed towards their terror of intimacy, but a black hole inevitably lies at the heart of every forensic assessment. We are dealing here with patients who may be consciously seeking to minimise or deny their acts of abuse. They may also be unconsciously defended against our attempts to think with them about the impact on them of their disability, their relationships with their primary carers, or their experiences of loss and separation. The risk assessment is not the place to remove such defences as there is rarely time enough to replace them with something more functional. We may notice what is wrong, but we are not seeking to treat it. This is the job of psychotherapy, or whatever form of treatment we are advocating. Risk assessment is the start of a narrative, not its conclusion.

CHAPTER THREE

When I grow up I want to have sex: working with children and young adults

In his 1912 book *The Kallikak Family: A Study in the Heredity of Feeble-Mindedness* the American psychologist Henry H. Goddard told the story of "Deborah Kallikak" a woman he worked with in the New Jersey Home for the Education and Care of Feebleminded Children (Goddard, 1912). Goddard had an interest in studying the origins of disability and, using Deborah as a case study, he traced her genealogy back to Martin Kallikak, her great-great-great grandfather, a Revolutionary War hero married to a Quaker woman. While still a young man, Martin had a sexual encounter with a "feeble-minded" barmaid that resulted in a son. Martin himself went on to become a respected citizen, head of a family of prosperous and successful children. Two branches of the Kallikak family tree were thus created: one containing disability and one without. Goddard concluded that the disabled branch, descending from the barmaid, was peopled by the insane, the delinquent, and the criminal, seemingly proving his hypothesis that "feeble-mindedness" was inheritable.

Goddard's conclusions were taken as scientific fact, adding weight to a eugenicist perspective that had a profound impact upon the way in which those with disabilities were viewed throughout much of the twentieth century. He was particularly interested in the criminality of the barmaid's lineage, seeing it as being fundamentally caused by intellectual disability. His book makes uncomfortable reading, conflating as it does disability and offending and describing children with disabilities as being inexorably drawn towards the perverse and the illegal. His work has been widely discredited, eschewing as it did any consideration of the social and economic factors affecting the failure of the "disabled branch" of the Kallikak family to thrive. The pseudonym Goddard chose for the family is an interesting indicator of his desire to split off the healthy from the perverse, as he coined the name from the Greek words καλός (*kallos*) meaning beautiful and κακός (*kakos*) meaning bad. For Goddard the young disabled offender is a product of his genes, his innate badness being immune to environmental or therapeutic change. Beauty is not allowed to flourish in this withered and dangerous branch of the family tree.

Much of forensic psychotherapy is concerned with the adult patient. For some patients this means that their treatment is a form of archaeology, with the analyst seeking to excavate into their histories to discover the aetiology of their perversion, what it was that was the genesis of their abusive behaviours. In this chapter I wish to examine the possibility of a more contemporaneous treatment—forensic disability psychotherapy with children and adolescents. I wish to consider afresh Goddard's thesis that disability and criminality are twinned by genetic imperatives, and to examine the role that forensic disability can play in the lives of children and adolescents who are seemingly bound to an unalterable trajectory towards adult criminality. In considering this I do not wish to restrict my thinking to working with young forensic disability patients from a purely diagnostic and investigative perspective; I wish also to examine this sphere of clinical work in a prophylactic context.

It has been estimated that approximately twenty per cent of all rapes and twenty to fifty per cent of cases of child abuse are perpetrated by children and adolescents (Barbaree & Marshall, 2006). Becker and Hicks (2003) delineate three types of young offenders:

i. Dead-end: Compounded by lack of education and awareness, young people who have committed acts of sexual abuse during their first explorations of sexual behaviour. The levels of recidivism are low for this type of young offenders.
ii. Delinquent: When sexual crimes form part of a wider pattern of antisocial and criminal behaviour.

iii. Deviant: Those young people whose psychosexual development is extremely disturbed, mostly by extreme trauma. This last group is most at risk of remaining offenders in their adult life (Ryan & Lane, 1997).

A range of studies have found a disproportionately high number of young sexual offenders have intellectual disabilities (Fyson, 2007). Vizard et al., in their early (1995) review of the literature on young abusers, found that forty-four per cent of referrals to a specialist clinic for young people who sexually abused others had some degree of intellectual disability, with half of these having attended a special school. Goddard and his followers may have been tempted to extrapolate from this that there is something implicit within an intellectual disability that preconditions someone towards acting out sexually. This is not the case. There is a disproportionately high number of young offenders with intellectual disabilities because there is a disproportionately high number of young victims with intellectual disabilities (NSPCC, 2003). While there is no absolute correlation between the experience of being abused and becoming an abuser, the victim-to-victimiser cycle has been shown to exist in a significant proportion of male perpetrators (though not among the female victims studied) (Glasser et al., 2001). Children and adolescents who commit sexual abuse tend to have highly dysfunctional family backgrounds, including neglect and physical abuse (Veneziano & Veneziano, 2002) with a high level of exposure to sexual and non-sexual aggression and pornography (Seto & Lalumière, 2010). Young people with intellectual disabilities who sexually abuse also figure more highly in the literature than their non-disabled counterparts because they are less skilled at denying or concealing their actions, and also tend to be more closely supervised (Fyson, 2007). Balogh et al. (2001) conclude that a key difference between young abusers with and without disabilities is that the gender of their victims does not matter to young abusers with intellectual disabilities. They are also more impulsive in their offending (Hackett, 2004).

Whether the child's primary traumatic experience is of sexual abuse, physical aggression, deprivation or neglect, the common denominating psychological experience of forensic patients is that of extreme powerlessness. In the most acute cases we see an intra-psychic fragmentation and incohesion, and a psychotic anxiety characterised by a persistent terror of annihilation (Hopper, 1991). Most young forensic patients are nearer than adult patients to the traumatic event or processes that they are seeking to gain mastery over through sexual offending. In treatment terms this is both good and bad. The relative closeness to the explosion of trauma means there can be more elasticity of affect. Traumatic symptoms have not been concretised and ritualised as they have for many adult patients. Neural pathways, while massively affected by trauma, carry more potential for change (Wilkinson, 2006). On the other hand, the young patient is much closer to the site of detonation, and carries with him the immediate, raw signs of damage.

The unconscious need to gain mastery over trauma by taking on the position of victimiser rather than victimised involves not just an identification with the aggressor. It can also involve an addictive, excitement-seeking edge. Alvarez (2003) highlights the need for therapists working with young abusers to share their understanding that the abuser abuses not just because he needs to, but because he likes to. She also describes the child's excitement at raping another child as stemming partly from his inability to feel ordinary excitement at ordinary pleasures. This is an important point, highlighting as it does the young forensic patient's displacement of pleasure into perversion. Trauma has blunted his capacity to feel alive. Sex or violence, or both, become the only tools the patient has at his disposal to fend off deadening annihilatory anxieties. Therapy with children perversely drawn to making others feel their humiliation, shame, and fear requires of the therapist the capacity to remain non-perversely alive in the face of deadening attack.

* * *

Quadir is seven, and has a mild to moderate intellectual disability, with some autistic features. He lives with his mother and his fourteen-year-old brother, who has been diagnosed with Asperger's syndrome. His school has referred him for psychotherapy, as one of the recommendations made in a recent risk assessment. On numerous occasions he has been discovered coercing both boys and girls to touch his penis. He has also been found putting his fingers into the vaginas and anuses of his peers. Prior to my first session with him I have met with his social worker, his teachers, and his mother, all of whom have conveyed tremendous anxiety about how to stop Quadir from growing into a serial sexual offender. His mother, in particular, has a dark cloud of anxiety floating over her, and I ensure that she is provided with psychotherapeutic support before my work with Quadir begins.

She accompanies Quadir to the clinic where I will be seeing him. As I sit in the consulting room I hear a clatter of something crashing to the ground, followed by Quadir's mother apologising profusely. It later emerged that Quadir had swept away all the papers that were lying on the reception desk before then running into the administration office of the clinic. He dashed to the filing cabinets, followed closely by his mother who grabbed hold of him just as he was about to upend a plant in the corner of the room.

As I come into the waiting room I see that Quadir is trying to destroy the various toys on the shelves around him. I introduce myself and ask if he's ready to come into the therapy room. He looks shocked, and then delivers a sharp kick to my leg. His mother apologises again, and I say that Quadir may be trying to let me know he's not sure if he feels safe enough to come into the room with me. Eventually he agrees to come in, as long as he can be accompanied by his mother. Once inside, he seems completely overwhelmed by the toys, puppets, and art materials that are available to him. He spins around the room, eventually taking an armful of dolls with him as he sits, crossed legged on the floor beside his mother. His play is frenzied, and he never seems able to stop and stay with any one toy for more than a few seconds. He grabs doll after doll, looks at it for a few seconds, and then throws it away, moving on without thought to the next one. When he has exhausted the dolls he moves on to the collection of small figures that are clustered around the sand tray. Later in the session he finds the paints and water, and delights in mixing them all together, forming a glutinous, multicoloured sludge that he stares at for a short while before pouring it over himself, to the horror of his mother. He then says he has to go, and pulls his mother out of the room.

I stare at the room. It is hard to believe that he has only been in it for twenty minutes at most. The level of mess looks as if it would have taken far longer and far more children to create. I am aware also of how the room mirrors my own feelings of messiness, my insides feeling as if they have been as shaken and mixed up as the paints. It is only now, in the aftermath of the storm Quadir unleashed, that I am aware of my physiological reactions to him. My heart is beating fast and my hands are shaky. I feel overwhelmed by exhaustion, and dread having to write up my notes about the session, fearing that I lack the capacity to make any narrative sense of what has just happened. I also feel inordinately worried, although it takes me a while to work out what specifically

I am struggling with. I am worried about his mother, how on earth she manages with the tidal waves of destructive energy her son unleashes around him. I am also worried about Quadir, as it is hard to see how he ever manages to stop and think, and how between us we will be able to create a space in which thoughts and feelings can be tolerated rather than forcibly evacuated by manic actions.

The work with him continues at this manic pitch for some months. I come to think of Quadir as being a kind of typhoon, spinning his way around the consulting room, chaos and mess trailing behind him. At first my main worries are about how the room and I can survive this weekly squall. Can I be the sturdy, storm-proofed structure whose foundations are strong enough to survive the tempest he personifies? Or will I be a flimsy, makeshift shack, my walls and ceiling being flung to the skies at his approach? At times the storm is sexualised. He grabs hold of his penis through his trousers, particularly when gazing at the dolls, squeezing his erection, and I am not sure if he is trying to stifle its potency or bring it to life. I see in this an unbearable juxtaposition of two sets of beliefs he holds alongside each other: one, that the world is a sexualised place, where there can be no boundary between one body and another, and where aggression inevitably finds its expression in sexually abusive ways; and Quadir's other, more shameful sense of himself, as someone who has to keep a tight grip on his penis for fear of losing it. Without this he is nothing; he may cease to exist. His sexualised rage is both violent and self-soothing.

Over time the storm abated. In one session he looked at me quizzically, raising an eyebrow as if to say "You still here?" I raised a smile at him and said "I'm still here. You haven't blown me away." After this, the storm came back sporadically, but it no longer had much strength to it. Instead of crashing into the room and filing through the dolls and toys in manic, unthinking ways, he began to hold them for more than a few seconds, brushing his fingers against different fabrics, as if beginning to notice that something could have a skin that could evoke healthy, non-abusive interest.

This came at around the time Quadir had been removed from his school after attacking a girl in his class. A new school had been identified, and I was in tense negotiations with them to try to ensure his psychotherapy could continue. The work was under threat, and there was a possibility that it could be snuffed out at any time. I have no doubt that Quadir picked up on my feelings of worry in the transference, and perhaps it was this he was raising his eyebrow to. I was still here, but maybe not for long. We survived this threat to the work, and he began to explore the walls of the room for the first time. He discovered a cupboard in which various toys were stored. He looked excited at this discovery and squeezed himself into a space between some cuddly animals. He then pulled the door to, shutting himself in. I was gripped with anxiety. Visions of him suffocating flooded my mind, and I said, loudly enough so he could hear, "Quadir, are you ok in there?" I could hear a muffled, "Umm" in reply, and then, "Like it here!" I realised there was no way he could suffocate, the cupboard having lots of gaps in the wood to let air in and out, and I moved my chair nearer to it, letting him know that I was moving so I could hear him through the cupboard door. I could hear a squeal of laughter at this, and then a low humming that continued for the rest of the session, until it was time for him to go.

The sessions began to assume a pattern. He would come in, do a brief tour of the room, checking that the usual toys were in their usual places, before popping himself into the cupboard, where he would stay until it was time to go. He would hum or sing to himself, and would also ask me if I was sitting near enough to the cupboard to hear him. Sometimes I would sit quietly in my seat, occasionally reminding him I was still here, and still thinking about him. A couple of times he asked if I would pick up one of the dolls and hold it, which I did. I remarked on what it felt like holding the doll—how soft its fabric was, and how lovely it felt to be holding it. He would then emerge from the cupboard, usually with a triumphant "Ta da!", to which I responded with joy, delighted to see him again.

Eventually he regained some interest in the room rather than the cupboard, with the difference being now that the room was able to be experienced as a containing environment rather than a target to be destroyed. He spent longer periods on the floor, picking out dolls to look at, often passing them over to me to comment on. One day I noticed that we were playing. Not in isolation, but together, with toys and dolls being passed between us, and him listening to me as intently as I listened to him. The school reported that Quadir had begun to regulate his aggressive behaviour more, and that they wanted to try some rudimentary psychosexual education work with him. I was relieved to hear their readiness to do this, aware as I was of his desperate need to know that bodies could be used in non-abusive ways, but feeling reluctant to break up the rhythm of the work we were engaged on together by doing this educative work with him myself. Instead I talked with the school about useful ways of doing this. Children with intellectual disabilities are much less likely to have access to sex and relationship education because of underlying resistances to view people with disabilities as sexual beings, scarcity of accessible resources, and lack of professionals qualified to provide the appropriate support (Sterland, 2013). This work became a valuable transitional space for Quadir, as he had begun to voice his desire to stop coming to see me. Saddened as I was by this, I had begun to get the feeling that he needed to experiment with engaging with the real world without the safety net of his therapy. He formed a good attachment to the clinicians engaged in his sex education work, and even managed to attend his final session with me, choosing to spend most of the time in the cupboard, humming and singing and, unexpectedly, whistling, a skill he had never exhibited before. It seemed a hopeful indicator of his capacity for growth, to show a new skill, a way of communicating that could be built upon in the future.

Quadir's need to place himself in the close confines of the cupboard, squeezing himself amongst the soft toys brought to mind Grandin's (2006) description of her life lived with autism, and the physiological and then psychological security she sought from close physical containment. Grandin designs livestock-handling equipment, one of her inventions being a body-glove type device that holds cattle when stressed and anxious. When she tested this device on herself, she experienced an extraordinary sensation of safety, with many of her autistic traits subsiding, to be replaced by powerful feelings of stillness and security. For many years Quadir was terrorised by fears of being contained. His mother's attempts to hold him left him feeling perversely uncontained, as if her embrace was an abandonment rather than a holding, evoking the manic oscillation between a need for fusion and a terror of engulfment that comes with the core complex (Glasser, 1979). He needed to create the holding himself, before he was able to transfer the responsibility for it onto his mother, via me. Perhaps the sound of my voice through the wood of the cupboard door activated primitive, infantile sensations of aural holding of the kind we can only suppose occurs in antenatal life. I became a transitional object, preparing him to encounter the consulting room as a microcosm of a safe, non-abusive world, before finally being able to encounter his mother as a secure maternal presence that can be stayed with rather than run away from.

Forensic disability therapy with children and adolescents must, like work with adults with disabilities, be attuned carefully to the developmental stage of the patient. There may be very little correlation between a patient's chronological and psychological ages, with most patients presenting with differing levels of developmental functioning according to the differing levels of trauma, stress or anxiety they are faced with. We can see from Quadir's case how many places in the spectrum he was able to occupy at different times. He was the infant, utterly unable to cope with the intrusiveness of the world, unable to internalise any sort of maternal reverie. He was the antenatal baby, needing to nestle inside the womb, to gather enough resources to emerge into the world. He was the curious seven-year-old, confused by sexual desires far beyond his developmental capacities. And he was also the adult—more than capable of taking up a powerful adult position in relation to his victims, the only position in which he could assume power.

In the face of the patient who transforms the consulting room into an approximation of their internal world, the need for the therapist to embody the secure base is paramount. My need to be the house that couldn't be blown apart by Quadir's typhoon calls to mind Cottis's (2011) description of her work with an adolescent girl with intellectual disabilities whose experiences of sexual abuse, neglect, and deprivation had resulted in a traumatogenic re-enactment in the consulting room. Nothing that Cottis could say seemed to quell her patient's sense of terror at being in the presence of someone who wanted to think with rather than abuse her. The girl, ill-equipped to introject the notion of a good maternal object, displayed a finely honed tenacity in her attempts to sabotage the work in a variety of aggressive ways. Her attempts to interpret her patient's terror of healthy intimacy having fallen on deaf ears, Cottis found herself repeating to her patient, "There are four walls, a window, and a door." At first her patient seemed as impervious to these words as she had to any other, and it was only after the constant repetition of the phrase in session after session, imparted with a soft, loving tone, like that of a mother cooing a lullaby to her baby, that the girl's aggression began to abate. "There are four walls, a window, and a door … four walls, a window, and a door …" This mantra, symbolising as it did the notion of a maternal object that could provide a psychological home, allowed this girl to locate within herself an internal object that could bear the presence of another. While the words were undoubtedly pivotal in their linking the parameters of the consulting room with the notion of an emotional home, Cottis suggests that her affect, the tone with which she voiced her mantra, the look of care and concern in her eyes, and the stillness of her body communicated as powerfully as her words that the room did not have to be destroyed, that it could become a space in which symbolic mothering could take place.

Much of Quadir's sexual aggression may be seen to be rooted in a profound annihilation anxiety. He had an impoverished internal landscape, thinly populated by internal objects that failed to provide him with the psychological nourishment he needed in order to thrive. The psychotherapeutic support given to his mother was fundamental in allowing him to experience her as a secure attachment figure with the capacity for thought and concern that became, over time, less vulnerable to being swept aside by her own anxieties.

Countertransference was key to understanding the motivations of this damaged and damaging little boy. Here I am thinking not only of how powerfully he projected his anxieties into me. They were also lodged very efficiently inside the clinic in which I saw him. The typhoon was not restricted to the consulting room, and continued to blow around the waiting room and the offices adjoining it for some months into his treatment. He came to occupy many of the thoughts of the reception staff, some of whom dreaded his appointments, resenting the pre-storm preparations they would have to make. Others spoke of him with more warmth, and, on occasion, love. Most forensic disability patients are stuck in a paranoid-schizoid position in which life is lived on a precipice. An ordinary feeling of sadness cannot be stayed with; it hurls the patient over the edge of the cliff into the oblivion of depression. A fleeting sense of joy is similarly indigestible, making the attainment of happiness, rather than manic, delusional ecstasy, an impossible task. This split between good and bad gets projected most powerfully into those working with children and adolescents because of the added potential for the enactment of parental dynamics. It is hard to be with a child or adolescent patient without being drawn into the vacant position of latent parent. The reception staff were so dramatically split between love for or hatred of Quadir because of the unspoken question lodged into all of them: how would we feel if he were our son? In the immediacy of the unconscious dynamic, "would", "if" and "were" are obliterated. We can only feel: "How *do* we feel? He *is* our son." In *As If*, Blake Morrison (1997) examines the trial of two children (Robert Thompson and Jon Venables) who killed another child

(James Bulger). For Thompson and Venables the game of ensnaring and torturing a child to death had no "as if" quality. It could not be a game that conveyed, "It is *as if* we are hurting you." It had to be concrete, a non symbolic play with deadly consequences. This captures the forensic dilemma, the patient's reliance on concrete thinking that masks an inability to think symbolically. Quadir could not stay with the symbolic. When faced with feelings of powerlessness, despair, and fear, he could not think, "It is as if I am dying. It is as if I want to hurt someone else to show them how badly I feel." He could only feel, "I am dying. I have to hurt someone else." And this lack of "as if" thinking was then projected into us, those situated around Quadir with all our human frailties, our vulnerability to taking in aspects of Quadir's paranoid schizoid, concretised thinking. It was difficult for those around him—receptionists, mother, therapist—to avoid falling down on one side or the other—love or hatred.

Woods (2003) takes an optimistic view of forensic psychotherapy with young people, seeing adolescence as a time of therapeutic hope before psychopathologies becoming too deeply ingrained and untreatable. I often found myself comparing Quadir with adult offenders I was working with who exhibited similarly worrying psychopathologies, but about whom I seemed to hold less hope. What was never known about Quadir was the genesis of his forensic behaviour. I came to think that it was rooted in extremely early object relations, looking to his positioning of himself in the cupboard and me outside the cupboard as his attempt to recreate and modify a parent/baby dyad. The consulting room was transformed from an arena of war and destruction to a place in which he could experience another as safe enough to be played with. It is doubtful that he could have managed this transition (or managed it quite so quickly) were it not for his retreat into the cupboard. I think his sojourn was a regression to the womb, a retreat from the chaos of a violent world to the safety of an oasis in which he could have complete power over his domain. There would be no impingements upon his sense of security, and he could maintain an umbilical link with me, a link that was both connector and communicator.

We have seen through the earlier chapters the need for forensic disability therapy to be practised in a systemic context. Nowhere is this more vital than when working with young forensic disability patients. These patients' lives are lived both at home and at school, meaning that school has to be as much part of the therapeutic team as parents, and a stable container for the work needs to be enforced to guard against splitting. Psychoanalytically informed treatment of the type described here cannot be the sole form of treatment available. Children and adolescents with intellectual disabilities tend to be far less informed about sexual matters than their non-disabled peers (Schaafsma, Stoffelen, Kok & Curfs, 2013), a factor that exposes their vulnerability to sexual abuse, both as victim and perpetrator (Servais, 2006). The primary aims of forensic psychotherapy are to facilitate the processing of trauma, build insight, and develop empathy. Forensic disability patients tend not to be able to access knowledge until there has been at least some processing of their primary or secondary trauma. Affect and cognition are interdependent phenomena, requiring for the young forensic disability patient a therapeutic model that can facilitate the development of both spheres (Greenberg & Safran, 1984). In Quadir's case it was not possible for the therapy to take on an educative agenda—the therapeutic space had to be too concerned with the processing of trauma, leaving little space for other areas of development to be accommodated. In other cases it can be more possible for the forensic therapist to take on the mantle of teacher, alongside that of therapist.

"Jamie", a twelve-year-old boy with moderate intellectual disabilities, had worked with Amy, his therapist, for just under six months. In her consultation with me, Amy explained how Jamie's history of neglect had begun even before he entered the world, his disability caused in large part by foetal alcohol syndrome. He had never seen his mother, as she had died of an overdose shortly after his birth. Since an early age Jamie had shown signs of severe sexual aggression, attacking other children in the various homes in which he had been placed. At the age of eleven he had raped and tried to strangle a girl in his class at school—a shocking case that had hit the headlines, giving him a certain notoriety and placing upon all those professionals working with him a fearful desire to get things right as the world was watching (several tabloids periodically ran stories on Jamie, usually dripping with rage that he was receiving treatment rather than punishment). Despite a difficult start during which Jamie refused to enter Amy's consulting room for six weeks, she felt she was beginning to get somewhere with him. He was particularly attached to sand tray therapy, in which he would pick out small toys from Amy's shelves and place them in a sand tray. Amy would then encourage him to make up a story, linking the toys together. Rather inevitably the stories tended to concern mothers leaving their babies, superheroes battling against super criminals, and invisible fathers.

In a recent session Jamie asked Amy if she had a penis, like him. Amy interpreted this as Jamie's desire to know whether she could understand what it was like to be him, to be a boy with a penis, and to be a boy with a penis that got him into trouble. In choosing to work with this within the transference Amy was working primarily within the affective domain, but neglecting the cognitive. She may well have been correct in supposing that Jamie was yearning to be reassured that he could be understood by her, but it was my sense that she was missing his other need to have questions answered about bodies and what they are for. Amy's initial response was to look at whether this psychoeducative work could be undertaken by someone else, as, much like my work with Quadir, she felt that the work was too cluttered emotionally to allow for something more educative to take place. I was of the opinion that she had to modulate her approach to accommodate both. To continue her work in understanding Jamie's relationship with trauma, while also allowing herself to answer some of his concrete questions about what body parts were for, what constitutes a boy and what constitutes a girl, and what to do with the rush of sexual feelings cascading around his body. Jamie had the capacity to relate to Amy as both an affective and a cognitive object. For other children this duality of role is too confusing, and they need to have their confusion addressed elsewhere, leaving their therapy free to bring their feelings about their confusion.

For forensic disability therapy with children and adolescents to work most effectively, it has to be located within a sturdy container. The disparate parts of the treatment package—psychotherapy, psychoeducative, parental support, school input—need to come together on at least a quarterly basis to review the progress being made in all domains. The potential for splitting is as strong as it is in adult forensic disability work. Perhaps it is stronger, given the heightened feelings activated when faced with a child who hurts other children. We tend to be comforted by the known and the familiar, and the stereotypical image of the sex abuser—the adult male stranger (strange, in every way)—exists to protect us from the disturbing implications of those forensic patients who are not adult, who are not male and who may not even appear to be strange. Children are meant to evoke love and care, and it can be difficult to access those feelings when the child is a sexualised, aggressive attacker. A powerful part of the splitting processes involves denial and dissociation, and the presence of regular meetings in which all those involved in the care of the patient come together can help to guard against the fantasy that all the work is being done by the therapist, relieving everyone else of anxiety and fear. These meetings have so many purposes—to share information, to assess risk and to plan future interventions. They are more basically a place in which the horrendous weight of caring for a child who has abused can be shared.

Our work with children and adults with intellectual disabilities has to be developmentally informed. Intellectual disabilities so powerfully affect the capacity to make the transition from one developmental stage to another. The moves from infancy to childhood to adolescence to adulthood all involve loss, and the need for mourning. We are working with patients whose problems in moving healthily from one stage to another may, in Wilber's (1984) terms be thought of as having a "developmental lesion", manifesting itself in particular forms of psychopathology.

Forensic disability therapy is about messiness: the mess of brains atrophied by trauma or starved of love, of boundaries that have to be compulsively broken, bodies that do not know where they end and another's begins. This disarray will inevitably have to find its expression in the consulting room. The bringing in of mess, conveyed through sand, water, paints, clay, or the "harmonious mix-up" (Balint, 1979) of all of them, is the patient's attempt to bring us closer not only to the world they inhabit, but also who they feel themselves to be. The mess we struggle to tolerate in the consulting room is an outpouring of early relational trauma, be it abuse or neglect (O'Brien, 2004), making it unsurprising that our countertransference responses are so often victimised ones. We are the containers into which all of our young patient's identifications with victim and abuser need to be evacuated.

Working with young forensic disability patients involves a mix of stillness and movement. The work will often be very physical, involving working at the child's level and being prepared to play alongside them. Alvarez's (2012) notion of the vitalising level of analytic work with children reminds us of the need to convey an affect-laden, enlivened, and enlivening interest in the patient whose experiences of neglect and deprivation have caused an atrophying of their interest in themselves or in others. At times this has to involve many aspects of the therapist becoming enlivened on behalf of the deadened patient—through the voice, the eyes, and, indeed, the whole body. At other times it can be as important to maintain a sense of stillness in the face of destructive attack. The child who feels himself to be a typhoon seeks to destroy the world in order to convince himself that nobody can survive him. It is a deeply sadomasochistic expectation that has to be countered by the therapist who can sit out the onslaught of the storm, that does not get blown away by the child's rage, enabling the child to finally meet someone who believes in creation rather than destruction.

Goddard was wrong to think that a child with intellectual disabilities is more likely than his non-disabled peers to become a criminal, simply because of his genetic code. To understand sexual perversion through the lens of DNA is to ignore the profound impact of trauma on the lives of the children and adolescents we work with. It is also a way of denying the presence of hope. If sexual crime is genetically determined, what is the point of therapy? There is a window of opportunity with young patients; the sooner we can intervene the less inevitable their journey towards life as an adult offender becomes. In working with young forensic disability patients we are working with those who are at the very centre of multiple experiences of traumatic and traumatising change, and who often lack the cognitive and affective capacity to form a narrative with which sense can be made of chaos.

CHAPTER FOUR

Speak no evil: the role of creative therapies in working with severe disability

The sexual abuse of others is the enactment of pathological depressions and anxieties that the perpetrator has been unable to put into language. Forensic psychotherapy is concerned with putting speakable words to unspeakable actions, to allow patients relief from inflicting the agonising narrative of their life onto others. While we tend to think of psychotherapy as primarily a talking treatment, there is a growing evidence base for its more creative methodologies in the forensic world, including art therapies (Smeijsters & Cleven, 2006). Most people with intellectual disabilities, even at the mild or moderate end of the spectrum, encounter difficulties with verbal communication (Iacono & Johnson, 2004), including speech that is hard to understand, problems in understanding what is said, and difficulties in expressing themselves because of limited vocabulary and sentence formulation skills. How much should this matter in the consulting room, given the traditional privileging of psychotherapy as the "talking cure"? When words are not the primary tool of communication, we need to look to the non-verbal. Mehrebrian (1971) concluded that just seven per cent of the communication we engage in on a daily basis is verbal (words only). Thirty-eight per cent is vocal (tone of voice, silence, inflection), and fifty-five per cent non-verbal. According to Argyle (2013) non-verbal communication is five times more influential than verbal communication—this research defining non-verbal as including facial expressions, touch, gestures, interpersonal spacing, and posture. In their study into how people with intellectual disabilities and severe communication difficulties signal their distress, Regnard et al. (2007) found a median of twenty-four changes in signs or behaviours per person, indicating that a wide vocabulary of non-verbal communication was able to be accessed and expressed by the supposedly "non verbal" patient. It is hard not to conclude from these findings that our psychotherapeutic reliance on words may be in danger of blinding us to a far richer discourse.

While we tend to privilege the idea that language is essential to human interaction, we often neglect the idea that the opposite is equally true (Goldin-Meadow, 2006). In making sense of the aetiology of a patient's disability alongside their capacity for language, we have to be mindful of the possible impact of trauma on the developing mind's ability to grow, learn, and develop. A patient's lack of verbal language is not always solely a consequence of a cognitive deficit. It may stem from early trauma—be it environmental or interrelational, or a mixture of both. Some of the processes involved in the expressive language delay of children with intellectual disabilities are associated with problems in an earlier nonverbal phase of communication development (Mundy, Kascari, Sigman & Ruskin, 1995), while others may be more clearly seen to stem from overt trauma such as the impact of maternal depression, the witnessing of domestic violence, or the experiencing of sexual abuse.

Patients with severe intellectual and/or communicative disabilities can disable us far more than patients with mild or moderate disabilities. One defensive structure we are liable to erect to fend off these disturbing feelings of disablement is to seek to put words into the mouth of our patient, to shield ourselves from the terror of not knowing by becoming all knowing. When the severity of a disability reduces the possibility of clear verbal communication, meaning should be viewed as the negotiated outcome of interactions, always involving inference, but remaining at heart an intersubjective process. Validity of interpretation is thus a continuous rather than a categorical variable (Grove, Bunning, Porter & Olsson, 1999), meaning that our function as partial translator of our patients' material is a truly dynamic and often confusing process that inevitably changes its parameters as the relationship between analyst and patient lengthens and deepens.

It is also possible to be so profoundly affected by the severity of our patient's disability that this becomes their main diagnostic feature—the signifier that identifies them to us, causing other nuanced aspects of their self to remain invisible. It is too easy for patients with severe disabilities to be subject to what Reiss et al. (1982) first termed "diagnostic overshadowing", the process by which clinicians are quantitatively less likely to diagnose symptoms of mental ill-health in patients with disabilities, as compared to non-disabled patients. The diagnostic overshadowing phenomenon diminishes the significance of abnormal behaviour, with clinicians seeming to ascribe the "abnormal" solely to the disability, rather than being interested in it as a symptom of trauma, abuse, or psychiatric instability. The tendency to ascribe all manifestations of pathology to the disability rather than to traumatogenic or environmental factors increases incrementally with the severity of the disability. Symptoms of trauma thus lie hidden within the disability, causing those with severe disabilities to be even more absent from the consulting room that those with mild or moderate disabilities.

Verbal communication involves the use of both signs and symbols. The sob in the patient's voice as he provides a narrative about his mother, telling us he is experiencing sadness, is a sign—a product of the emotion it signals. But it is the symbolic content of communication that accounts for its extraordinary effectiveness. Regardless of the type of signal, all communication involves the transfer of information between one person and another, making it a profoundly intersubjective phenomenon. Working with forensic patients with severe disabilities requires a close attunement to the symbolic level of communication. While not exclusively the domain of severe disability (it is also an issue occurring in the analysis of those with mild and moderate disabilities), time has a particular symbolic meaning in the analysis of patients with severe disabilities. The intensity of the analyst's interest in and curiosity about them may be too rich a diet to digest, meaning it has to be consumed in bite-sized morsels. What remains important in such cases is the analyst's capacity to bear the full fifty minutes, even if forty-five of them are spent in solitude. The fact of the analyst's declaring they will stay thinking about the patient, even if the patient needs to leave the room before their full time is up, may eventually induce the patient to experiment with joining them for longer stretches of time. Even if it does not, however, it remains an important indicator of the therapist's refusal to collude with the patient's notion that he is worthless and should be ejected out of the therapist's mind as soon as he is out of the therapist's sight, as we will see in the following vignette.

* * *

"William" fills his institution with fear. He has lived in their care since he was two, when his parents were forced to acknowledge they were unable to care for him any longer. Thirty years have gone by and he still carries the raw wound of this loss, as if it had been inflicted the day before. He is a tall, thin man who looks both young and old. At times he can seem like a child, skipping around the building, searching for games to play, filling the air with the song he loves to whistle, over and over again. At other times he can feel far older to the staff working with him. On days like these he wakes with great trepidation, as if the world is a dark, foreboding place, with catastrophes waiting to hit him. William has severe intellectual disabilities. Due to a series of hospital failures, his brain was starved of oxygen at birth, leaving him with a terribly diminished capacity to talk. He can manage words of one syllable and no more. Various speech and language assessments have pointed to a disparity between his expressive and his receptive language skills, with most professionals concluding that he can comprehend more than he can express. His mother has described him as being a baby who was, literally, "hard to handle". He tended to scream for most of the day and most of the night, rarely responding to any attempts to soothe or comfort. He was the youngest of six children, and it surprised nobody when his parents made the painful decision to place him in local authority care after a couple of years in which their emotional and practical resources were thinned and stretched to breaking point. They continued to visit him every weekend, up until the death of his father, when William was eight. Acting on the advice of friends and professionals, William's mother decided not to tell him of his father's death until some months after the funeral had taken place. In that time she had sought to prepare him for the worst by letting him know his father could not make the visit that day because of "feeling poorly". William reacted to this with confusion, although it is hard to tell how much the confusion was caused by his difficulty in processing this painful information, and how much it was magnified by the confusing and disturbing feelings he was picking up from his mother. As hard as she worked to suppress her own grief, it leaked out as soon as she sat down in the institution to play with William, suffusing their interactions with an unacknowledged but powerfully felt sense of unexpressed mourning. The confusion was exacerbated by the sudden absence of William's siblings, who were barred from visits because of the fear that they would blurt out the news deemed too painful for him to hear.

It was around this time that William was taken away by his institution for a week to a holiday camp. It is suspected that during this week he was sexually assaulted by an older boy with disabilities with whom he shared a room. Based on the experiences of other children who later disclosed their own abuse at the hands of this boy, it is thought that William was anally raped, and forced to perform oral sex. Staff at the time noticed a sudden deterioration in William's behaviour. He became unmanageable, seeking to trash his room, physically attacking other children, and constantly seeking to abscond from care. The holiday was deemed a failure, and was the last break from the institution that William had for many years, as it was thought that his attachment to the familiar space of the institution was too great for him to tolerate any changes in environment.

With puberty came the onset of aggression, as if a violent time bomb had finally been detonated. William began to lash out at all those around him, punching members of staff and attempting to strangle other service users. A special assistant was delegated to accompany him everywhere, with the dual task of protecting others, and also providing him with an experience of a safe and supportive relationship, something his increasingly difficult behaviour prevented him from accessing from others. His mother struggled with dealing with a son who showed so much aggression and so little compassion, and over time her visits diminished in frequency. William began to be fixated on other children's genitals, and was found on numerous occasions trying to touch both boys and girls in their private parts.

William's adolescence and early adulthood were times of deep confusion for him, in which his sexualised aggression was able, at times, to be managed, but which tended to become his default position when faced with any kind of external stress. William's mother died when he was twenty-seven, an event that overwhelmed him completely. A form of almost catatonic depression fell over him like a shroud, and for two years he withdrew from the world, remaining in his darkened bedroom, responding to nobody apart from his sister, the only sibling who had continued to visit him from childhood. In the past few years he has begun to emerge from his depressed shell, due largely to the efforts of "Janet", a play therapist employed by his home to see him at least three times a week.

Janet was brought into the home following a particularly brutal sexual assault that William had perpetrated upon a cleaner in the home. She had attempted to get him to move from his bed so she could remove the sheets for washing. Her efforts to coax him out seemed to serve only to heighten his rage and his anxiety, to the point where he grabbed hold of her, pulled her into the bed with him, and started to feverishly touch her private parts. She struggled free from him, but was traumatised by the attack, eventually leaving the setting because of her fears of being assaulted once again. A risk assessment was conducted, and it was recommended that some form of therapy be sought for William, alongside a tightly constructed risk management programme which would reduce the likelihood of him being alone again with a potential victim.

Janet spent the first eight months with William negotiating with him the possibility of their having a shared therapeutic space. He was accompanied down to her therapy room, and, while his escort worker sat unobtrusively in the corner, she watched as William began to form a relationship with the room. At first he would stay for, at most, five minutes. He would occasionally sniff one of the toys in the room, or poke his finger into the sand tray, before running to the door, mumbling "bed—bed", meaning that he wanted to return to the safe cocoon of his bedroom. Janet would comment on his retreat, reminding him that she was going to stay in the room while he went to his bedroom, and she would continue to think about him, even though he hadn't stayed in the room.

It was around this time Janet found herself feeling overwhelmed by her work with William, and struggled to retain any sense of hope that she could ever be anything more than a shadowy presence in the room, someone who William would only acknowledge as much as he could acknowledge that there was a chair in the room, or that the walls were blue. In supervising her work, I wondered with Janet about this void, empty countertransference that threatened to shut down any possibility of her connecting with William. She described considering handing in her notice, as it no longer felt ethical to claim money for simply waiting in an empty room three times a week. I wondered what did actually go through her mind while she sat there, alone. Janet thought long and hard, and eventually replied, "I don't think about him, in the way I tell him I do. I don't hold him in mind, to use the cliché. I think about how I'll get from the centre to my next appointment, what the traffic will be like. Sometimes I think about my children, and how they are, especially if they've not been well the day before. But that's the normal guilty working mother stuff. And eventually I find myself feeling guilty, really guilty. For taking money for nothing. And for being so useless. I wonder what the staff must think about me, sitting here, all on my own, doing nothing."

We began to disentangle what was Janet's, and what belonged to William. How much of the hopelessness and shame was part of Janet's internal landscape (a question partly answered by comparing the weight of these feelings with their absence while working with other, less disturbed patients), and how much was being projected into her by William. Our supervision sessions moved from an analysis of what was or was not going on in the consulting room, to a more free-floating exploration of what might be going on in his internal world. This allowed Janet to relieve herself of some of the pressure of the projections that had been evacuated into her, providing us with a more creative space in which to place ourselves inside William's imagined mind. The feelings of uselessness held by Janet were eventually understood as emanating directly from William's sense of being worth nothing, of having a life that appeared to mean nothing to anyone or, worse still, appeared to be a burden to others, a drain on the resources of all those around him.

As Janet began to sift through and separate the interwoven fragments of her and William's interpsychic experiences, he began to stay in the room for longer periods, to the point where he reached what seemed to be his natural limit of thirty-five minutes. Within this time he seemed to learn to experience Janet as a form of auxiliary ego, an external voice box that could articulate suggestions, questions, and wonderings about what he was making of the space they shared. He began to form an attachment to the small toys that he tended to bury in the sand tray. They were a disparate group of animals, family figures, and superheroes, their common denominating factor being the fact that they all ended up buried, heads down, in the sand and were left there, without a backwards glance, by William as he left the room at the end of his session. Over time he began to be interested in Janet's interest in the toys, and her wondering about both what they represented for him, alongside the significance of how necessary it seemed to William to be able to abandon them at the end of each session. While, at first, William could not tolerate Janet's interest in him, causing him as it did to shut down, or to run out of the room, her interest in the toys seemed to allow him to consider interest as something potentially benign. Eventually he began to be interested in Janet, with the beginnings of a rudimentary dialogue becoming embedded within their relationship. He rarely used words, and when he did they tended to be "bed" or "sleep". Janet echoed these words back at him, sometimes infusing them with a life that was absent from William's dry, dead monotone. In one session she found herself increasingly disturbed by his tonal deadness, and took a strange, unexpected risk: she began to sing the words back at him. "Bed!" she sang, stretching the word out luxuriously, letting her voice modulate up and down the scale, creating a harmony from the single syllable. She did the same with "sleep", and both songs evoked surprise and astonishment in William. He stared at her for some time, allowed himself a tiny smile, and then repeated "Bed" back to her, eliciting yet more singing from her. This became a feature of the sessions, assuming a maternal quality, with Janet becoming the good enough maternal transference object in whose company William could begin to play—an activity it is hard to imagine him ever learning to do in his actual childhood.

With play comes growth and change, not least in the domain of the countertransference, which it should not be assumed will remain maternal, just because it may have started with these qualities. When working with severe disability, the countertransference becomes the primary map with which we navigate the patient's internal world. That which cannot be held in mind by the forensic patient tends to be projected into the mind or, indeed, the body of the analyst. The erotic transference is a frequent if under-discussed component of the forensic project. Mann (1999) makes the point that there are as many variations on the erotic transference dyad as there are analytic couples, and, of course, that there are many differing perspectives on what the erotic transference symbolises and how best to work with it. The move of Janet from a maternal to a sexual object was a subtle transformation, and one that initially filled her with what Kumin (1985) describes as "erotic horror"—an overpowering sense of foreboding about the depth of William's feelings of longing for her. It should be noted that this process was only obliquely raised in a supervision session when Janet described noticing how, when waiting for William to be brought to the consulting room, she shifted her chair back a couple of inches from its normal position, creating a sense of distance between her and him. In analysing the reasons for this stepping back from the powerful intimacy between therapist and analyst, Janet talked for the first time about her growing feelings of fear about being in the room with William, despite the presence of the member of staff, and her anxieties about him attacking her within the session and, more potently, her sense of violation at the idea that she had become a masturbatory object to him. "Bed" had taken on a new meaning for her, and she found herself becoming more reluctant to sing it back to him, as if the maternal cooing had been replaced by a siren song of desire and invitation. The maternal attunement and infantile need that had seemed to link them in a benign way had been replaced by an "erotic bond" (Mann, 1994)—a suffocating and overwhelming tie that had been woven as a result of a heightened activation of erotic material in the unconscious. We worked together on how best to—using Wrye and Welles' (2013, p. 87) phrase—"tolerate the heat without fanning the flames" of the erotic transference.

Janet's continual question of me in our supervision was "Is this really therapy?" She was attuned to the non-therapeutic quality of the institution in which this work was happening, and often found herself imagining the shock that William's care staff would feel if they knew how little "real therapy" she was doing. Her anxieties clustered particularly around the member of staff who was in the room throughout the sessions and, despite this member of staff's protestations that she could see the unfolding of a truly therapeutic process, Janet continued to fantasise that she was secretly harbouring all sorts of cynical and judgemental thoughts about what she was witnessing. My response to Janet was "It's therapy, but not as we know it"—a reminder of the need to broaden one's creative parameters when working with forensic patients who are at the more severe end of the disability spectrum. It was my view that this piece of work was profoundly psychotherapeutic in its orientation. Janet was working in the transference—a particularly deep maternal transference that was allowing early object relational material to be accessed and worked through. She was working within well constructed therapeutic boundaries, and holding on to an understanding of the unconscious as being absolutely key to an understanding of the conflation of intrapsychic anxieties that had served to create William's perverse and aggressive sexual enactments.

The other side of the erotic transference coin is the dead or deadening transference. When working with severe disability we are often encountering moments of deadness, moments of life-draining boredom that threaten to kill off any capacity for reflection and life within the work. The sessions can have an awful circularity, with patients wanting or needing to go over the same limited material over and over again, with seemingly little change or development in either the material they are repeating or their ability to think about it. Phillips (1993) describes boredom as being either a form of depression—a kind of anger turned inward—or a longing for that which will transform the self. Fenichel (1955, p. 295) delineated two states of boredom: one a quiet, languid state, the other a state of fidgetiness, while Wangh (1975) linked boredom with an alteration in our relationship with time: "Time seems endless, there is no distinction between past, present and future. There seems to be only an endless present." (p. 541). Thus boredom presents an impasse to fantasy life, as fantasy is enlivening, the opposite of boredom. And play is all about fantasy. Boredom may also be seen as an unconscious resistance to disavowed longing, arising from conflicts about libidinal fantasies, and aggressive wishes. Brenner (1974) suggests we approach boredom as if it is a symptom, always asking what conflicting forces bring about its formation. Embedded within the boredom we feel with the severely disabled patient may be a desire to kill him off, to relieve us of the agony of sitting with the bleak emptiness of his mind and the slow, hollow tedium of a lack of mental reciprocity. We are throwing coins into a well, and rarely hearing the reassuring splash as they reach the bottom. Instead there is silence.

When working with patients whose level of disability is manifest in an overarching deadly boredom that threatens to engulf both patient and analyst, we can be helped by Alvarez's investigations into finding and tuning into the right analytic wavelength (Alvarez, 2012). In describing work with psychotic patients Bion (1957) described making contact with the "non-psychotic part of the personality", a concept Alvarez has built upon with her work with children with autism, in which she is interested in the different gradations of autism that are present in the patient's mind, implying an equivalent non-autistic part alongside the autistic. In approaching the child with the right band of intensity she has formulated a level of interpretation that seeks to vitalise the deadened state of mind. This stands apart from the two other levels she has identified as being explanatory/locating or descriptive/

naming interpretations, levels of interpretation that fit more neatly into classic notions of analytic neutrality. What Alvarez is describing is a form of interpretation that recognises the need for something more enlivening, something that acknowledges the atrophied and deadened aspects of a patient's psyche, and that seeks not only to wake these parts up, but which also reminds the patient that the analyst has not been deadened by the boredom of the disability. She is interested enough to want to bring something to life.

As is the case with many forensic patients with severe disabilities, the work with William involved the presence of an escort in the therapy room. The introduction of a third person into what is primarily a dyadic process carries an inevitable potential for confusion, splitting, and boundary breaking. In this case the "third" is present in order to guard against potential danger. In other cases they may be required, particularly in the initial stages of the clinical work, to help the highly anxious patient acclimatise to the new and threatening environment of the consulting room—a transitional object that can help the patient regulate his fears of entering an unknown and potentially overwhelming terrain. Another function of the third is to act as a translator, someone who can interpret to the therapist the patient's individualised language, be it sign language, use of symbols or articulation of grunts and groans. Phillips (2000) writes about the aim of psychoanalysis as being to free people to translate and be translated, saying, "people come for psychoanalysis when their present language no longer works" (p. 130). Many patients with severe disabilities have never voiced a language that has been truly understood, and have often resorted to violence and sexual aggression as a futile attempt to voice both their frustration at being untranslated, as well as their violent hatred of the world that cannot seem to decode their encoded narrative.

An act of translation also needs to happen with the "translator"—the third person in the room for whom psychotherapy may be an arcane, baffling, and threatening language which, if not made sense of, may seem to them to be nonsensical, useless, or dangerous. This requires of the forensic disability therapist a willingness to provide a map for the third person, some form of guidance about the territory that psychotherapy may cover, alongside a glossary of the language of the unconscious. Without this, it is likely that the third person will either seek to sabotage the work because of their misreading of it, and their sense it has no real value for the patient, or that they may become overly traumatised by the process. Being in the presence of a psychoanalytic process cannot be equated to simply watching a performance unfold. The third person is far more than an audience; she is, potentially, as much a part of the therapeutic process as the two other players in the room.

Forensic psychotherapy is concerned with fantasy; the patient will rarely be immune to an ongoing wondering about who the therapist really is. Even before transferences emerge, forensic disability patients are particularly susceptible to paranoid fears that their therapist must hate them—not only because of what they have done, but more centrally because of who they are. The oxygen of the consulting room is thick with paranoia and a constant fear of failed dependency. Most forensic patients have already had an experience of parental failure and it seems inevitable to them that this will be replayed again. It is inevitable that the third person will be the subject of fantasy—by both patient and therapist. The need for pairing (Bion, 1961) can cause both to wonder who the third person is allied to. These dynamics may also assume an Oedipal quality, with the patient caught up in an unconscious desire to kill off one object and pair with the other. It is important that as these dynamics emerge they are identified through interpretation so that their potential to be acted out (by any part of this analytic triangle) is diminished. There needs to be an explicit acknowledgement of the real, as opposed to the symbolic presence of the third. They exist in the room in the pursuit of safety or the facilitation of translation. Their introduction in the room presents both risk and possibility.

I have found psychoanalytic thinking the most useful container of my work with forensic disability patients, but I am also mindful of the need for other, more creative methodologies when working with those at the more severe end of the spectrum. Play therapy is traditionally considered as being suitable solely for children, although it has been demonstrated to be equally suitable for a wider age range, from babies and very young children (McMahon, 2009) to the elderly (O'Connor & Schaefer, 1994) with toys being shown to hold a myriad of symbolic meanings for patients with severe disabilities (Brodin, 1999). It is a developmentally sensitive intervention that requires of the therapist an attunement both to the chronological age of the patient, the functioning age and, most importantly, the developmental stages that the patient may regress to and from during the course of treatment. Play-based techniques are useful in assessment of patients prior to treatment (Gil, 2011), and are techniques that can be practised by those other than the therapist. McMahon (2009) explores the delineation between play therapy, as practised by therapists, and therapeutic play, as used by a wider range of professionals for whom its function is not psychotherapy, but the facilitation of a growth in trust and safety between patient and professional. Therapeutic play is also of use in working with patients in the pre-therapy stage, for whom participating in psychotherapy provokes too much anxiety, and who require a period of playful holding and containing work before they feel more able to give informed consent to entering therapy.

Sand tray therapy is a powerful medium for use with patients, regardless of verbal ability, but is particularly useful when working with those whose receptive skills outweigh their expressive. The use of paints, clay or other tactile materials can allow patients to make mess in the consulting room—a mess that may equally be a symbolic representation of their own internal sense of themselves as full to brimming with untouchable, unlovable messiness, or an evocation of the messiness of their perversion. It is far from rare for the forensic disability patient to quickly become attuned to any trace of revulsion or fear in their therapist. Their psychic antennae will be alive to any bats' squeak of hatred of their disability, their perverse symptomology or, more fundamentally, their core self. The therapist's capacity to withstand the outpouring of mess in the consulting room functions as a barometer of the parental transferences evoked in the work. Is the psychotherapist a mother/father who can withstand being saturated with the disarray of the disabled self? Will they be drowned by the weight of chaos being poured over them or will they be able to hold a safe and containing boundary that can allow the mess to begin to be thought about? Will their capacity to assume the mantle of quasi mother/father in the analytic work be diluted or destroyed by the mess they have to wade through, or will they themselves become as disabled as their baby? When working with patients for whom words are not the primary language, these questions are encoded within the transference and countertransference, requiring at some times a transference interpretation but, more often, requiring of the therapist the strength to hold on to these profoundly disturbing and potentially debilitating countertransference responses within their mind.

This level of creative work, aimed at allowing mess to be held and transformed within and between patient and therapist, has a particularly powerful function in enabling non-verbal early experience to become known. Artwork created within therapy has been shown to activate neurological structures of the brain, with mess itself being seen to be a consequence of damaged neural pathways resulting from early relational abuse (O'Brien, 2004). The faecal, visceral quality of working with clay, paints or water can allow the forging of a new relational paradigm in which the therapist is experienced as someone who can bear to hold the ambivalence of severe disability—the love alongside the hatred of the child, and all it can or cannot do.

Communication problems can be profound, even when the patient uses words. The problem can sometimes be a surfeit rather than a deficit. It was some months into a therapy with a forensic patient (who I will call "Derek") with mild to borderline intellectual disabilities before I realised that his telegraphese way of speaking was stopping any real communication from happening between us. Take this excerpt from the beginning of a session (which should be read with the knowledge that Derek's voice had a metallic, monotone quality to it—a voice that was difficult to read emotion into or from):

> "I saw my brother in that café where I had the—he said about his job because they're letting people—and Jenny said not to worry about it all because if I keep on worrying and worrying and—I've got this pain in my leg again—and then the bus was late again."

This gives a flavour of how this patient would flood each session with a string of unfinished sentences, while I sat, often unable to claim my space in the session. Sometimes the sentences would, in fact, be related to each other, but often if they were, it was inaudible to me. What helped was thinking about his way of speaking as being representative of his view of himself, to the point where I was able to say, "I think you don't think what you say matters enough, that's why you don't let yourself finish your sentences. But, you know, it *does* matter, and you *could* finish them. I'd really like to hear more than the first half of what you're trying to tell me." The impact of this was almost immediate, with Derek noting that I disagreed with his deeply internalised view of himself as someone who did not matter, who deserved to present himself to the world as a stream of broken pieces.

Derek's way of speaking—preventing a linguistic exchange between he and I—was also an attack on turn taking, that most fundamental human activity (Lepper & Riding, 2006). Schegloff (1992) describes turn taking as the practical manifestation of intersubjectivity, with its roots in the early development of the self, and I came to view Derek's scattergun approach to speech as being an echo of his early object relational history. His unconscious refusal to allow the two of us to "turn take" reflected an aggressive defence structure with which he could shield himself from the threat of intimacy. The more he could fend off the notion of a shared dialogue, the safer he could feel in his unreachable isolation. He oscillated between symbolically attacking me with his confusion of tongues, rendering me unable to think and to commune, and retreating completely from the possibility of a relational exchange. He demonstrated that aspects of the core complex (Glasser, 1979) can be manifested as much in the communicative as in any of the other domains.

Working with severe intellectual and/or communication disabilities requires of us a capacity to privilege the non verbal over the verbal, with much of the transmission of information and affect between patient and analyst taking place within the countertransference. Just as the patient's traumatogenic narrative can be seen as a triumph of actions over words, forensic treatment necessitates a reversal of this pathology, so that, even if the patient continues to lack verbal language with which to make sense of their perverse actions, the analyst can both hold in mind and give voice to an ongoing translation of all that has been encoded into silence and action. While not exclusive to the domain of severe disability, the erotic transference can have a particular potency when working without words, given the forensic patient's struggle to view others as anything other than sexual objects. Psychotherapy with forensic patients with severe intellectual and/or communication difficulties involves a broadening of parameters, with creative techniques being an invaluable addition to the therapeutic lexicon, enabling both analyst and patient to find new ways of giving voice to the unspeakable. When working with forensic patients with severe disabilities, the potential for the analyst to be subsumed by boredom is a constant risk, with the deadening effect of tedium serving as a defence against the threat of sexualised aggression emanating from the patient, or a murderous intent stemming from the analyst, or a toxic mixture of both. It is with such patients that Alvarez's notion of finding the right analytic wavelength acts as a form of symbolic lifebuoy for both players in the analytic dyad, allowing an aliveness to be experienced, and a therapeutic connection to be created.

CHAPTER FIVE

The disability transference: transference and countertransference issues

The narrative of forensic disability psychotherapy is largely constructed in the "here and now" experience of the countertransference relationship. Through an intersubjective exchange of feelings, thoughts, and memories a jointly authored narrative emerges that is guided as much by affect as cognition. The countertransference becomes the repository for those elements of the patient's unconscious he cannot bear to keep hold of, providing the therapist with projected aspects of the forensic patient's self and allowing an insight into those aspects of their perversion that can rarely be put into words. Through this process the countertransference becomes an invaluable tool with which the patient's internal landscape can be mapped and navigated. In this chapter I wish to examine various theoretical concepts relating to transference and countertransference in forensic disability therapy. Through examining some clinical vignettes in which failures to work through problematic transference issues have resulted in breakdowns in therapeutic functioning, I will outline the notion of the disability transference, a way of conceptualising the various countertransference implications of working with patients with disabilities.

Working with the countertransference in forensic disability therapy requires of us a capacity to encounter and engage with the most grotesque enactments of perversion. We find ourselves on the receiving end of projective processes that all too easily feel more concrete than symbolic and which can fill us with a horror that has the power to shut down thought. When faced with the risk of violence in others we must face the risk of violence within ourselves, just as working with sexual aggression requires of us the courage to acknowledge our own internal pockets of perverse thought. When the option of flight from the consulting room is unavailable, the inevitability of fight must be faced. Being in the presence of someone who has carried out acts of sexual abuse upon another human being means being attuned to countertransferential responses that may range from the healthy to the perverse: horror, fear, murderous rage, disbelief, prurience, excitement, and arousal. Projective processes are intensified when the alleged perpetrator has a disability, as we must then also process our desire to abort, ignore, and hate the patient, personifying as they do our repressed fears of our own internal disabilities. While some clinical trainings may alert us to the primacy of the countertransference in working with forensic patients, it is difficult to be prepared fully for the collective power of working with the abused, the abuser, the disabled, and the disabling.

Transference was first understood by Freud as an unhelpful form of resistance to being analysed. It was seen to occur as a result of unsatisfied libidinal need, compelling the patient to seek attachment to the analyst (Freud, 1912b). Freud later amended his views to encompass the notion of transference as a necessary and useful element of psychoanalytic work, and it is this latter notion that continues to resonate in a more contemporary view of the usefulness of transference and, indeed, of countertransference. The Kleinian understanding of countertransference has been summarised by Hinshelwood (1999) as being rooted in the *specific* response to the patient and not in a non-specific neurosis of the therapist. The therapist serves as a container for the experiences that the patient is unable to withstand and containing these unbearable experiences leads to the therapeutic mechanism of translating experiences into words. A pathological countertransference is the failure of the therapist to comprehend when the patient begins to resemble an aspect of the therapist that the therapist still has not learned to understand. Different types of countertransference have been described by Ryle and Kerr (2002, p. 104) as personal countertransference (what the therapist brings to the encounter) and elicited countertransference (the reaction induced in the therapist by the patient), the latter being either identifying or reciprocating. In the following vignette I wish to examine the interface between these two notions, the personal and the elicited, in order to consider the particular contours and colours that working with the perverse, disabled patient bring to the countertransference.

* * *

"Colin" is referred for risk assessment following a series of sadistic sexual attacks on children. He is in his early sixties, has a moderate intellectual disability, and lives in a group home, along with three other men with intellectual disabilities. His team describe him as "difficult to like", and it is clear that this stems not just from his abusive actions. "There's just something about him," says one of his workers. "Not something you can put your finger on. Something, I know it's wrong to say, something about him gives me the creeps." This impression is heightened by his appearance. He has lank and greasy hair and a grey pallor that suggests more death than life. His verbal communication skills are poor. His grammar and syntax are often difficult to decipher, but he is able to form a narrative that can be understood by another.

Little is known about his early life. He is an only child. It is thought that his father left his mother early on, and his mother died when Colin was around ten. He then moved to the care of his grandparents, who died when Colin was in his thirties. He was placed in the first of a long series of homes, his sexual compulsions making most of them untenable. He has a feverish compulsion to masturbate, and has been known to spend many hours engaged in an addictive, relentless form of self-abuse. His grasp of physical boundary is poor, and he has been known to take out his penis in public, with little or no regard for the feelings of those around him. He hoards pornography, mostly adult and mostly heterosexual. His first known abuse of a child occurred in a shopping centre, when he absconded from his escort and was found in a toilet cubicle forcing a nine-year-old girl to masturbate him. Despite the high level of supervision and monitoring afforded him, this was the first in a series of assaults—mostly in public places. Colin has been cautioned by the police on a number of occasions, but the fact of his disability seems to have rendered him immune from criminal charges.

My first session with Colin begins with him shaking my hand. Just before he entered the room I had been re-reading some reports on his compulsion to masturbate, and as his hand touches mine something inside me shudders and I feel a wave of revulsion towards him.

He is obese, and dressed in a tracksuit that has the look of a babygrow, adding to the sense that I am in the room with a barely grown up infant. He sits down, and I seek to ascertain how much he knows about me, and why he is here. He launches straight into a description of his "bad habit", as he puts it. He tells me he "can't stop wanking", adding that it doesn't matter where he is, he has an unquenchable desire to masturbate, a desire that no one has ever helped him to manage. The detail with which he describes his masturbation is extraordinary. He talks about having masturbated that morning in the kitchen of his home and in the toilet of the train that had brought him to the session. His eyes are glassy as he relates this and his breathing laboured, and I ponder on the masturbatory relish with which he is telling his story. I ask about other things that have gotten him into trouble and he tells me about the children he has abused, segueing into these descriptions with apparent ease. The session seems to be a quick one, and as we run out of time I remark on how much he has shared with me and wonder how he is feeling now. "Good," he says, and smiles.

I realise afterwards as I sit down to write up my notes that I can recall very little of all that he has shared with me. I jot down a few notes about his appearance and the handshake but I soon grind to a halt. I recall him saying such a lot, but little of it has lodged in my mind. This phenomenon repeats itself the following session, despite my determination to focus more acutely. He fills the room with his body and his words, but very little seems to stay with me, as if there is a barrier between us blocking the transmission of thoughts. Either this, or my mind has become sieve-like, unable to contain my thoughts about Colin beyond the time that he is seated before me. Feelings, on the other hand, *do* get transmitted, and I try to focus more on recalling these. It is hard not to concur with his team's sense of him as someone for whom it is hard to feel warmth. I realise as the sessions progress that I dread seeing him, often hoping for a call from his home saying that they will have to cancel the appointment. I am forced to recognise that I feel strong antipathy towards him. I hate his presence in the room. He has a stale, mouldy smell, and after he leaves I throw the windows of the consulting room open wide, seeking not just to expel his smell, but all trace of him. His physicality seems to oppress me and I find myself shying away from his attempts to get close to me, to shake my hand, or even to stare into my eyes. He feels too invasive, evoking in me a fear that the smell of him is getting into the pores of my skin, threatening to contaminate and toxify me. I hate the way in which he describes his masturbatory compulsions and his abuse of children. I fantasise about cutting the assessment short, saying that I feel I have enough information to conclude what his level of risk is and what risk management strategies need to be implemented to ensure children are safe from him. The thought of seeing him for ongoing psychotherapy appals me, although his team reports that he seems to have formed a good attachment to me and has spoken with them about whether he can see me once the risk assessment has come to an end. I realise as I reflect on this case with my supervisor that I dread getting to the end of the assessment without having learned anything about Colin beyond my hatred of him.

One of Winnicott's great gifts to psychoanalysis was his underscoring of the importance of recognising, without undue guilt, the role of hatred in the countertransference when working with severely disturbed patients (Winnicott, 1949). Just as a mother has to tolerate her hatred for her baby without doing anything about it, I had to find a way of holding my hatred for Colin without enacting it through killing off the assessment, aborting him before he could come to term. Colin embodies many of the countertransferential qualities that make forensic disability therapy so challenging on a particularly personal level. When faced with someone whose disability touches on our own primal terrors of being disabled, it is unsurprising that we wish to abort that fear by aborting them. In order to work with a patient with intellectual disabilities we have to work with our hatred of the trauma they personify. Trauma comes from the Greek word for wound, and in working with disability we are being brought terribly close to a wound that we desperately wish to disavow. Our patients bring into the consulting room a visceral embodiment of damage, injury, and impairment, evoking unconscious fears that the wound is contagious, and that, by our closeness to the disabled patient, we run the risk of losing our capacity for thought and intelligence as well.

The forensic transference

Those moments in session with forensic disability patients when the analyst loses the capacity to think, to remember, and to communicate stem from the conflation of two separate but related intrapsychic phenomena. First, there is the forensic response. Our patients have committed the most horrific crimes against the most vulnerable people. Our job is to help them recall the barbaric details of these crimes and to form a narrative that can make unconscious, perverse compulsions more amenable to conscious regulation. The act of sexual abuse breaks down the barrier between thought and action, rendering every thought the forensic patient has as being potentially catastrophic. If the desire to sexually abuse a child cannot remain in the realm of fantasy, the patient faces an unenviable struggle to know where thought ends and action begins. There is within this phenomenon a highly complicated grief reaction, as the patient struggles to process the move they have made from the normal to the abnormal. In leaving the world in which thoughts remain thoughts and not actions, the patient has not only entered a world without the containment of boundaries, they have also joined the world of their own abuser. In this perverse universe the patient has to deal with the pull of so many conflictual drives: the sexualisation of loss, the wish to gain mastery over their status of victim by assuming the role of victimiser, grief for the loss of the non-perverse self, and murderous self-hatred. The act of sexual abuse fuses the internal abuser with the internal abused, setting in place an inter-psychic conflict that cannot be borne alone by the patient. The split has to be evacuated into the therapist, who is then experienced, through a form of projective identification, as a fused object: seduced and seducer, lover and abuser, prisoner and imprisoned.

The forensic psychotherapist is thus involved in a profound transference relationship in which the defence mechanism of splitting is activated by the patient in order to fend off the depression they are psychologically unequipped to feel. The location for much of this splitting is within the countertransference, with the therapist acting as the container for the patient's unfeelable feelings, such as depression, sadness, love, hatred, arousal, and numbness. Contained within my countertransference responses towards Colin was a sadistic attitude. My hatred towards him found a home in fantasies about cutting short the assessment, refusing to shake his hand, or humiliatingly drawing attention to his personal smell. As Temple (1996) points out: "A perversion involves a sadistic attitude towards the object, who can respond in a retaliatory fashion, and so be sadistic in return to the patient, or become masochistic and accept the role of victim." (p. 35). Transference and countertransference phenomena are particularly problematic in forensic psychotherapy because of the intense disturbances embodied by the forensic patient, and the primitive defences erected to fend off thought and feeling. Moving on from this wider notion of a forensic transference, I wish now to consider the notion of a disability transference that has an equal, if not more powerful, impact upon the work.

The disability transference

In working with intellectual disabilities, countertransference is affected not just by un-analysed parts of the therapist's neurosis, but also by the therapist's relationship to his own disabilities. Freeman observed a preponderance of guilt, anger, over-sheltering, over-identification, overestimation of abilities, and co-dependency with patients (Freeman, 1994). While Freeman's studies were into therapists whose disabilities were diagnosed, and thus explicitly known to the analyst and, on occasion, to the patient, I am interested also in thinking about us all, patients and therapists alike, as existing somewhere within a spectrum of disability. Being in the presence of a patient with a disability forces us into an encounter with those parts of our own psyche that resonate with notions of lack and loss. Just as it would be extraordinary if an analyst working with a patient with a missing limb did not find himself reflecting on what his own life would be like without an arm or a leg, it is unsurprising that when working with patients whose minds have been slowed or damaged by congenital or environmental factors—trauma or injury—we find ourselves imaginatively occupying their psychic space. Just as the tongue is drawn to the missing tooth, our thoughts cluster around missing cognitions in an attempt to both reassemble what is missing and to imagine how we would live with such a lacuna.

Countertransference is not just a theoretical construct; it is an affective phenomenon that has the capacity to aid our understanding of our patient's internal world while also holding the potential to cause harmful enactments. Under the pressure of countertransference feelings arising from both patient and therapist the therapy itself is at high risk of becoming disabled. In her study of cognitive analytic approaches to working with patients with intellectual disabilities, King (2005) notes the temptation on the part of the therapist to deny the presence of disability in their patient, leading to a lack of connection with what is, and has to be, real in the consulting room. Segal (1996) noted the propensity of some therapists working with patients with disabilities to unrealistically limit their expectations of what therapy may achieve, based largely on a prejudicial view of the patient's ability to tolerate painful emotions.

Aragão Oliveira, Milliner and Page (2004) focused in particular on the impact of a patient's physical disability upon the therapist, linking distortions judging the patient's prognosis with the therapist's own castration anxiety. Levitas and Hurley (2007) discuss countertransference as a factor in the over-medication of patients with intellectual disabilities. The patients they studied were being medicated in direct proportion to their caregivers' fear of them, rather than as a result of any quantifiable diagnosis. Here can be seen an alarming disparity between the real issues presented by a patient's violence and a separate neurotic response to it, leading to an enactment of an uncontained countertransference response. Drawing on psychoanalytically oriented group psychotherapy with severely physically disabled patients, Watermeyer (2012) has examined countertransference responses to both the impaired mind and the impaired body, linking universal unconscious conflicts evoked by impairment to a need to place those with disabilities out of society's sight. The lens through which we seek to observe and assess our patients with objective neutrality is thus sharpened, focused or unfocused by the emotional experience of sitting with the disability of another, resulting in an impasse caused by unconscious countertransference attitudes in the therapist that remain unaddressed. As Segal puts it most succinctly, "counter-transference is the best of servants but the worst of masters" (1986a, p. 86).

Disability therapy requires of its practitioners a capacity for what Keats (1817) called "negative capability"—"when a man is capable of being in uncertainties, mystery, doubts, without any irritable reaching after facts and reason". It is, of course, a fiction to suppose that one human being can ever know another fully. Bion's approach to psychoanalysis made use of his capacity for "not knowing" (Bion & Rickman, 1943), thus creating space for thought and meaning to grow and develop in more reciprocal ways. The Symingtons (2002) elaborated Bion's approach in their warning of an overly investigatory analytic approach when "intolerance of the unknown and our need to snatch at something that 'explains' it smothers the opportunity of coming to the truth" (pp. 182–183). The Bionic stance of privileging not knowing over knowing is particularly challenging in disability therapy. Patients come with a hunger to know, having spent their lives in positions of enforced unknowing, their cognitive deficits making it hard to hold and process knowledge and information. Faced with this hunger, a maternal transference quickly develops, magnifying a countertransferential response of wishing to nourish, to give knowledge to the unknowing, to feed on demand, thereby disavowing the necessary developmental experience of frustration.

We may consider there to be two types of split emotional reaction to working with the trauma of disability: excessive involvement in helping the patient and showing empathy with them, or, on the other hand, avoidance of and distancing from the problem personified and carried by the patient. These have been differentiated in characterological and clinical terms as the traumatofilic and the traumatophobic therapist (Wilson, Lindy & Raphael, 1994). There is considerable risk at both ends of this countertransference spectrum. The traumatophobic forensic disability therapist whose responses are overly coloured by hatred of their patient's crimes, dispassion for his history of trauma, and contempt for his attempts to elicit empathy is bound to fail his patients and be tremendously vulnerable to vicarious traumatisation. The traumatophilic therapist who can only attune to the victimised part of their patients, shying away from any exploration of their sadism, hatred, or perversion will find himself similarly caught up in a therapeutic failure. One of the most seductive failures within forensic disability therapy occurs when an overly protective parental countertransference is enacted, causing a blurring of boundaries that echoes the patient's own valency for eroding and breaking the limits between their subjectivity and that of another.

* * *

"Tom" was referred to Jenny, an experienced psychotherapist. He was in his late twenties, and had Down's syndrome. He had recently been moved to a new group home, having been evicted from his previous home following allegations that he had sexually assaulted two younger men with disabilities. Jenny had been recruited by the new home to provide him with individual psychotherapy as part of a risk management strategy designed for them by a forensic psychologist. At first the work seemed to go well. Tom was highly motivated to attend his sessions and reported feeling understood by Jenny. She in turn enjoyed working with him, finding herself genuinely engaged in helping Tom make sense of a chaotic childhood history littered with sexual abuse and emotional deprivation. He seemed particularly engaged in using creative therapeutic techniques. Jenny, who had trained in art therapy, was pleased at how well he used drawing to articulate a family narrative that he struggled to put into words, and she found herself buying more art materials for the consulting room. Tom noticed these materials, and asked if he could take some of them back to his home. At first Jenny felt uncomfortable about the request, but came to see it as evidence of Tom's desire to introject something good from the therapeutic work, and eventually gave him a set of finger paints to take home from the session. At around the same time, she began to find it increasingly difficult to end the sessions on time. Tom invariably seemed to be in the middle of an engrossing piece of artwork when the time came for the session to end, leading to Jenny gradually extending the sessions, by a couple of minutes at first, and eventually by ten minutes.

At Christmas Tom gave Jenny a picture he had drawn at home; it showed them both in the consulting room, surrounded by pens, pieces of paper, and crayons, beaming widely. Jenny was delighted by the gift, and, in answer to Tom's questions as to where she would put it, she assured him she would take it home and find somewhere "just right" for it. Tom became ill with flu over the Christmas break, and said he felt too low to attend sessions in January. Jenny suggested she visit his home to ensure that the therapeutic work was not disrupted by his illness. A staff office was hastily converted into a therapy space and, from then on, a pattern emerged of some sessions still taking place in Jenny's consulting room, with a growing number of sessions taking place within Tom's home.

One of the most striking elements of this vignette is how little of it was ever discussed within supervision. The time incursions were never brought up by Jenny, mainly because she had experienced me as being, in her view, overly rigid about boundary issues, and felt that I would not accept what she saw as the validity of Tom's desire for more time with her. Kelly and Wadey (2012) describe two main types of boundary phenomena that occur in forensic mental health settings: insidious and high impact boundary testing. *Insidious* refers to the kind of daily chipping away at boundary that can occur in wards and group homes—patients gathering personal information from professionals while having a friendly chat, the professional gradually disclosing more and more information and, under the guise of reciprocity and benign availability, becoming over-involved with the patient. This insidious boundary testing often goes unnoticed, with a new, unboundaried way of relating becoming the accepted norm until things begin to gradually slip out of control. Kelly and Wadey differentiate this from those *high impact* boundary tests that tend to be more visible and which require limit setting in the face of threats, intimidation, or violence. In this case, the insidious boundary testing ultimately gave way to a high impact test. A family crisis caused Jenny to have to redraw her time boundaries with Tom, meaning that she could no longer let sessions overrun. Tom responded in their next session by attempting to sexually assault Jenny, an assault she narrowly avoided by escaping the consulting room and calling for help from staff.

The attempted assault was the culmination of a complex set of transference and countertransference phenomena that had caused action to replace thought, in potentially catastrophic ways. In analysing the situation some months on from the attempted assault, Jenny was able to identify a blind spot in her countertransferential responses to Tom. He had evoked in her an overwhelmingly maternal response of a particular colouration. He had become to her the child who had to be fed on demand, who could tolerate no frustration and to whom terrible things would happen if she put limits in place. At the heart of this was her response to his intellectual disability and, more specifically, to the fact that he had Down's syndrome. Jenny described having always felt a tremendous empathy towards people with Down's syndrome, a tendency to view them with sympathy, and a reluctance to think of them in any negative light. This represented a colossal failure of analytic thinking, disavowing as it did the requirement of all forensic disability therapists to consider the role and function of hatred in the countertransference.

Tom had projected into Jenny his need for an all-gratifying maternal object, a transference figure he sought to entrap in a sadomasochistic dynamic whereby she was compelled to feed him on demand, with sexual assault being her punishment should she fail. He was unequipped to deal with the metaphorical loss of her breast, with sexualised aggression being his only response to this cataclysmic wound. His disability had been used by Jenny to soften the rough edges of his perverse symptoms, to the point where all she could see, hear, and relate to were those parts of him that had been abused, deprived, and broken. In her own way she had become as vulnerable to splitting as he had, being able only to disavow the bad in favour of seeing the good. His response was similarly split. The return to normal time boundaries was impossible for him to think about. Her taking back of his time was experienced not just as a removal of her love—it was a castration of him, an attack on his phallic power that had to be responded to with the potency of a sexual attack.

Jenny had become disabled by the power of the countertransference. Thought had been eliminated in favour of feeling, and the projective power of disability, underscored by the power of her patient's forensic symptomology, had robbed the psychotherapy of its potential for metaphor. Its exchanges had moved from the symbolic to the concrete, in a mirroring of the forensic dilemma, from painful thought to painful action.

* * *

The disability transference is a phenomenon that affects the capacity of the therapist to process thought. It is not just a cognitive process, occurring as it can also do within the "body counter transference" (Orbach, 2003). This can be thought of as similar to Krystal's (1978) notion of the "re-somatisation affect" in which transference and countertransference contents are enacted on the non-verbal level, affecting both body and mind. Common countertransferential responses in disability therapy include difficulties with making sense of narrative, time confusion, heightened somatisation, and impaired ability to communicate. Within the disability transference a number of complex processes are unfolding:

1. Projective identification
   The patient's disability is projected into the therapist, impeding thought and reflection.
2. Disavowal of hatred
   The therapist's hatred of the patient's disability is repressed, sublimated into a compensatory idealisation.
3. Disavowal of love
   The therapist's hatred of the patient's disability is over-privileged, allowing no space for a less split, polarised view of him as a human being rather than a disabled object.

The disavowal of hatred and of love should be viewed as interrelated processes that do not necessarily follow a linear trajectory. A therapist can oscillate from one response to another from session to session, and from moment to moment within one session. The disability transference takes as its cornerstone the notion that disability is a trauma, an event that cannot be naturally assimilated and processed, and that has the power to disable the therapist in a variety of unconscious ways. Thinking about trauma requires the capacity to symbolise, and, in order to be able to symbolise something, one must first finish grieving it (Segal, 1986b), thus moving from the paranoid-schizoid to the depressive position. Failures in disability therapy tend to stem from a failure on the part of the therapist to process the trauma of the disability, responding to it in a paranoid-schizoid, and thus a split, way. Concrete action replaces symbolic thought. A key determinant of a traumatic event is that the victim is unable to think about the event. Thinking about the event becomes the event. It cannot be processed and assimilated, leaving trauma with limited places to go in the psyche. As Britton states, it can be suppressed or split "into psychosomatic dysfunction, perceptual hallucination or symptomatic action" (Britton, 1998). Intellectual disability is a trauma, both for those parents who carry the weight of toxic shame about what their intercourse has given birth to, and the patient who both introjects the parental shame and thickens it with his harsh superego.

All exchanges between therapist and patient carry the potential for the therapist to fall prey to powerful transference and countertransference processes, diluting the potential for thought to function as an effective therapeutic agent. Sleepiness, failures to retain thought, and temptation to act rather than think are all manifestations of the disability transference, requiring the ring-fencing of a supervisory space in which the invasive quality of disability can be analysed and processed. There are cases, and Jenny's was one of them, where supervision is not enough, and a return to personal psychotherapy is indicated. This is most likely to happen within the domain of forensic disability therapy, where the combined weight of both the forensic and the disability transferences can become too much for the clinician to bear.

One can see, through a close reading of Jenny and Tom's vignette, how the power of the forensic and the disability transferences were intensified by the beginnings of an erotic transference. For Tom, the line dividing maternal from sexual longing was paper-thin, and his desire for Jenny was suffused with erotic longing, making her perceived rejection of him an intolerable humiliation on a number of levels. The erotic transference in forensic disability therapy can include a longing for an equal relationship with the therapist, a yearning for a merger in which all differences between therapist and patient are erased. At its heart this is a desire for the removal of disability. The patient longs to have their cognitive lacks taken from them, allowing them to be loved for who they are rather than what they are not. There will always be an unchangeable difference between therapist and patient. This can function as a form of trauma membrane (Lindy, 1985) in which the patient stays with the impossibility of being understood by someone who has not had the same traumatic experiences as them.

The challenge facing the forensic dyad is how to face the grief of non-reciprocity. The therapist has to fail the patient. This can best be considered in the context of the idealisation of the therapist, the placing of them into the vacant position of the maternal object who can provide reparation to the patient for the wounds suffered in childhood. The idealising transference (Kohut, 1971) communicates, in part, the patient's need to maintain a narcissistic fusion against feelings of emptiness and powerlessness. The imperative to satisfy the patient's desires is tremendously seductive. The patient's desire to be rid of their disability touches on profoundly painful aspects of the countertransference: the shame we hold about being the non-disabled part of the disabled dyad, and the guilt we feel about being unable to do anything to reduce the agony imposed upon the patient by the weight of their disability. Idealisation turns to denigration when the impact of the therapist's failure to rid the patient of their disability is experienced fully. The good mother turns transferentially into the withholding, perverse object who has to be disavowed, hated, or attacked. For the forensic patient, this leads to the activation of the core complex (Glasser, 1979) in which the patient's unconscious desire to merge with the therapist evokes a primitive fear of the intimacy this would involve. An almost inevitable lacuna in the psyche of the forensic patient is, of course, the ability to hold a healthy sense of intimacy. When faced with the intimate merger they hold both longing for and terror of, their response is to either withdraw into a state of autistic withdrawal, or to attack the object of desire. Glasser's concept is both a way of understanding the mechanics of perverse, sexually aggressive attacks, and of conceptualising the intricate movements of yearning and fear that reside within the transference and countertransference between therapist and patient.

Transference and countertransference issues are not confined solely to the domain of psychotherapy. If we embrace Sullivan's (1953) reading of transferences as "parataxical integrations" that occur in a far wider set of human interrelationships than simply the therapist/

patient dyad, a broader psychosocial understanding of the complexity of relationships between those with and those without disabilities may be gained. There are complex unconscious dynamics involving power and agency imbalances in most dyads where one person has a disability and the other does not. Power is both a concrete reality as well as a transferential dynamic. The forensic disability patient comes to the consulting room having lived a life devoid of power, ready to experience the clinician working with them as yet another embodiment of a disablist, disempowering society. The only attempts the forensic patient has made to exhibit power and control tend to have been perverse enactments of sexual aggression—the main reason for them entering the consulting room in the first place. While the desire for autonomy and control is rarely straightforward, more often being deeply equivocal and underpinned by ambivalent drives (Schneider, 1998), we cannot avoid the need to consider carefully the role of power in both the transference and the countertransference. Whether we side with Habermas's view of psychoanalysis as an emancipatory practice (Lichtman, 1990) or the Foucaultian view that the analyst cannot avoid participation in societal power dynamics in the consulting room (Guilfoyle, 2007), the relationship between a therapist and a patient is inherently unbalanced in terms of power (Boyd, 1996). The client traditionally travels to another person's place of work, that person controls the time, the frequency, the physical location, and the layout of the room in which the activity occurs. This power imbalance is writ even larger when the patient has an intellectual disability (Marks, 1999; Varughese & Luty, 2010).

* * *

The countertransference is the most powerful therapeutic tool available when working with forensic disability patients. Our capacity to be disabled by our patients provides us with insight into what it is like to have a mind that sometimes simply does not work. The interface between a patient's disabled and perverse selves adds weight to the projective power of the transference. We are inevitably vulnerable to a pull to act rather than think, to attack rather than maintain boundaries, and to become mindless rather than mindful. These drives are projective in nature, evidence of the unconscious' indomitable capacity to communicate through affect what words cannot convey. The deadened, atrophied minds of many of our patients are powerful signifiers of defence mechanisms erected to protect against the pain of disability. Better to not think when thought opens one up to depression, unbearable anxiety, and the agony of a life shrunken by disability.

I have used the notion of the disability transference to try to describe a phenomenon that has its roots in projective identification and can be used both as a diagnostic device and as a therapeutic tool. Working with the disability transference cannot be a solo venture. In dealing with the destructive potential of perversion and the deadening weight of disability, we are opening ourselves up to the destructive and disabled parts of ourselves. As Nietzsche wrote, "Whoever fights monsters should see to it that in the process he does not become a monster. And if you gaze long enough into an abyss, the abyss will gaze back into you." As will be explored in Chapter Eight, the supervision of forensic disability cases is far more than the provision of clinical governance. It is a protective membrane that enables us to be mindful of the seductive allure of boundary blurring and breaking, and the pitfalls of allowing our thinking to become softened or deadened by exposure to mindlessness.

CHAPTER SIX

Grieving the imagined baby: on working with families of forensic disability patients

"John" and "Rita" sit slumped on the couch. They are in their mid-fifties, but look much older. They appear stricken with anxiety, and I try to break the tension by asking about their journey here today. "Tough," says John, his voice heavy with exhaustion. "Really tough." It is clear he is talking about a far longer journey than the one I had in mind, so I invite them to tell me more. They take some time to settle into their narrative, with lots of pauses, silences, and anxious looks at each other, as if willing the other to carry the weight of their story. It is too much for one person to bear. Eventually the words come tumbling out and, while Rita is markedly quieter than John, there is a palpable sense of relief from them both in finally being able to put their story into words.

They are here because of "Maureen", their thirty-two-year-old daughter. Maureen has Down's syndrome and a moderate intellectual disability. She also has a long history of stalking mothers and babies, and recently kidnapped a three-month-old baby girl from outside a shop. When she was found, the baby's nappy and clothing had been removed and there were signs that she had been vaginally penetrated by Maureen. After initially denying taking and abusing the baby, Maureen admitted having taken the infant so she could "play with her, just like I play with my dollies." At the time of this meeting, the Crown Prosecution Service is deciding whether criminal charges will be brought. While John and Rita understandably want to begin with this most recent event, I encourage them to tell me more about how Maureen came into the world, and what her childhood was like. Rita describes her as "a little poppet", the culmination of a dream. They had had three sons before, and Rita had always yearned for a girl. John concurred with this, describing the joy when they discovered they had a daughter. The joy was short-lived as it soon became clear that she had Down's Syndrome. When I ask how they felt on being told this, Rita starts to cry. "It didn't feel real. I mean, we loved her. We've always loved her. But there was this dread. This horrible feeling that she'd never have a normal life. That she'd never be able to do what the boys could do. Never get married, never have kids." John adds, "And we worried about what would happen to her when we weren't around. Which is a crazy thing to think when your baby's just so young. But we couldn't stop thinking—who will she have when we're not around?"

They talk me through the first years of Maureen's life, and I am struck by how profoundly different it is from the normal tales of a child's development—the thrill of the first word, the move from crawling to walking, the pain then the pleasure of the first tooth. In place of these moments of joy is the recounting of a kind of war, a war of endless battles: the battle to find the right school for her, to find childcare for her, to take her on holiday in places where she would not feel stigmatised and stared at. "She was always conscious of being different," explains John. "And by then we'd pulled ourselves together, you know? We've moved on from that initial shock, and we loved her so much, always wanted the best for her. And it was hard when you came up against prejudice. When other kids didn't want to know her, or other parents talked about her like she wasn't there, saying terrible things, really, I suppose not meaning to be cruel, but saying things that made us feel like everything about her was wrong."

They describe noticing her sexualised behaviour from the age of four. "She'd put her fingers into her private parts, almost like she was trying to comfort herself. But it never stopped; she never grew out of it. And then she'd always be really interested in babies—always had such a fascination with them. We didn't think too much of it, until she was about seven, and we found her with our neighbour's baby, with the baby's nappy taken off." Both John and Rita break down at this point, as they describe the beginning of a long history of sexual enactments, usually against babies or small children. Their battles with the world continued, as they struggled to work out why Maureen was so drawn to babies, and why there was such an alarming sexual edge to her interest. Despite endless consultations with social workers, psychologists, and psychiatrists, no answer was provided.

At twenty Maureen moved into a group home for people with intellectual disabilities, a move that filled them both with much guilt. "It was the right thing," says Rita, "I know that. We weren't coping. We couldn't cope. But it always felt like the worst thing we could do, as well." Through her twenties Maureen veered from one crisis to another. Her weight ballooned and she was put on strong antidepressants as the team around her struggled to cope with her increasing volatility. At times she was violent, lashing out at members of staff and attacking other residents. Other times she regressed to a childlike state, crying for hours about wanting to be home with her mother, wishing to see her brothers. "The boys have always been good with her," said John when I asked about Maureen's relationship with her brothers. "They find it tough though. One of them can't have anything to do with her now, not since he had children. And the other two are patient with her, but she wears them out. She can lash out, and she can make them feel absolutely terrible. Not as bad as with us, but bad enough."

As our meeting ends, I ask John and Rita what they hope for now. There is a long and heavy silence, and both of them look blankly at me. I am suddenly aware of a powerful countertransference response in me—a feeling of guilt at introducing to them the abstract notion of hope. As carefully chosen as I hope they are, my words still seem to have the capacity to render these two people mute with grief. "I don't know about hope," says John, at last. "We hope, I suppose, she'll get some sort of treatment. That they can find some kind of way to stop her doing these things with babies. But, beyond that, I just don't know. I wish everything was different, that's the truth, and it can't be." Rita sobs, and says no more. We end, and as he is leaving the room John seems brighter and says, "It was good to say it all, I suppose." Rita nods, and I see the beginnings of a small smile, something that instantly lifts her worn, tired features. "Yes," she says, "it had to be said." After they go I find myself unable to get on with other work for quite some time, affected not just by the overwhelming power of their story, but also needing to process my response to the glimpses of hope that they expressed on the edge of the session.

* * *

One act of sexual abuse has many victims. We can see here how Maureen's actions have traumatised her parents in a profound way. They are not just two depressed and traumatised individuals. They personify something we see in so many forensic disability cases: a deeply depressed, traumatised, and disabled family. The trauma is not located solely around Maureen's abusive actions. It is located too in far earlier trauma—her birth, and the realisation that she will not fulfil the hopes they held of a healthy, "normal" daughter. Sinason and Osborne (1993) describe the aftermath of the birth of a child with disabilities in traumatogenic terms, mapping out the initial shock and ultimate sense of loss as the yearning for the "perfect" child is dashed, leading to high levels of depression in parents of children with intellectual disabilities (Olsson, 2001). Cottis (2009a) uses an attachment-based perspective to consider the notion of disability as a traumatising factor within a family, affecting not just the parents, but the siblings as well. I would add to this Bálint's (1979) notion of the "basic fault" in the bio-psychological structure of every individual, involving in varying degrees both mind and body. Bálint traces the origins of this fault to the early formative period, during which serious discrepancies arise between the needs of the individual, and the care and nurture available to them. John and Rita's narrative can be heard on two levels—the object relational and the forensic—and our job is to attend to the overlap between the two.

In thinking with them about their experience of hoping for the perfect baby I was struck by how they were describing an experience of primary loss in which the fantasised child they had held in mind during the pregnancy had seemed to die, to be replaced by the feared, disabled child. In her descriptions of "conceived fantasies", Raphael-Leff (2001) explores the ways in which pregnancy can be a time of dreams and nightmares, fears and fantasies, infusing the mother's waking and dreaming states. The imagined baby is the receptacle of so much expectant imagining, an astonishing process of two people living under one skin. The overlap between the intrapsychic and the external feeds anxiety, as society's tendency to regard the disabled child as "less than" has a powerful impact upon all mothers. In my work with Irish mothers of children with intellectual disabilities, for example, I have been struck by the fact that the most common phrase said to them by those struggling to acknowledge their child's disability was, "I'm sorry for your troubles," a phrase used more commonly when commiserating with someone about the death of a loved one. And it is in this linguistic salve that we can see something profound being acknowledged—that the birth of disability can be experienced as the death of the imagined, healthy baby. (Here I am using "healthy" in the same way that mothers use it when they say they don't mind whether their baby is a boy or a girl, they just hope it is "healthy".)

The death of the imagined baby is an invisible, unwitnessed death for which there are no containing rituals through which mourning can be facilitated. In describing their realisation that Maureen had Down's syndrome, John and Rita spoke most strongly about their shame, fed both by their sense that they had done something wrong to ostracise them from the "normal" world of happy parents with non-disabled babies, alongside their ambivalence towards their helpless and vulnerable daughter. Their first container of shame, that something about their union had disabled their baby, echoes Sinason's (1992) use of Wolfensberg's (1987) phrase "death-making" to describe the unconscious fantasies held by patients that their disability has been caused by something deeply destructive in their parent's intercourse, making damage instead of love.

To be able to talk about one's love and hate towards one's baby remains one of the most deeply embedded parental taboos (Parker, 2005), making it difficult for either parent to speak about their disappointment, their wish that their tiny, helpless, dependent baby had a mind that worked normally, and a body that did not look so different from the bodies of others. In working with John and Rita, all three of us became interested in exploring how these primary feelings of disappointment were magnified by Maureen's visible appearance of disability. They described feeling "branded" by how different Maureen looked from other children, meaning that moments when her disability could be ignored by others were rarely, if ever, available to them, as they might be for parents of children whose intellectual disability has no physical manifestation. Just as issues of physicality and embodiment were worked with in Maureen's own psychotherapy, the notion of her core identification with difference stemming not just from a brain that was disabled but also by a body that advertised her sense of otherness was an important one for John and Rita to consider and process.

It became clear that Rita experienced profound postnatal depression following Maureen's birth, with John's work making it difficult for him to provide the kind of emotional support she needed at the time. He too was depressed, although he learned to manage it in different ways, mainly by throwing himself into his work, creating a necessary buffer between his sense of self and his feelings about his disabled daughter. These dynamics are not exclusive to parents of forensic disability patients, residing more widely in families where sexual abuse has not featured at all. I call this the *primary parental trauma*, and suggest it requires special attention be paid to how the parents have experienced the birth of the child with disability, and what therapeutic support is necessary to ensure they do not become stuck in a state of pathological mourning. In this, the primary loss seems never to have been mourned, resulting in a life lived in a perpetual state of depression and melancholy. With John and Rita we are also seeing the effects of a *secondary forensic trauma*. They have been further disabled by the knowledge that their daughter is sexually excited by babies. This knowledge has reduced their capacity to think, as it has compounded the original unprocessed primary trauma. They have never mourned the imagined, non-disabled baby, making it hard for them to now mourn the imagined, non-abusing child.

What is required in this and similar cases where neither the primary nor the forensic trauma have been processed, is a psychotherapeutic intervention that will enable the facilitation of a long delayed and multi-layered process of mourning. Just as Maureen required a thorough assessment of her psychological capacities before deciding what level of psychotherapy she could make best use of, parents and families need to be assessed with an equal amount of thought and sensitivity. John and Rita proved themselves able to use an intervention that was, basically, psychotherapy. Despite the years of struggle they had survived, they had retained a capacity to think and to reflect and were, in many ways, hungry to start processing the trauma with which they had lived for so long. Other families are nowhere near the state of psychological preparedness that John and Rita demonstrated.

It is clear that forensic disability therapy is an intervention that cannot exist in isolation. It is as much a systemic as it is a psychoanalytic project, and where the family is the system, we need to examine the level of therapeutic intervention that they can bear and that they can make use of. Clarity as to what the aims are of such work is essential. Is its primary goal to develop insight? If so, there are cases where the family matrix is too cluttered with anxiety-driven dysfunction and trauma to allow space for real reflection. There are other cases where insight is too threatening to admit, particularly where perverse family structures dominate or where there is a risk of adult psychotic breakdown. Rustin (2000) formulated a spectrum of parental support in mainstream child psychotherapy which took as its guide the level of emotional capacity demonstrated by the parents. I wish to adapt this model for use with forensic disability cases

Level 1	*Educative*
Methodology	Providing advice and information, avoiding, as far as possible, insight-based interventions
Frequency	Monthly
Primary aim	Protecting and sustaining the forensic patient's therapy
Indicators of suitability	Resistant to support, dysfunctional, enmeshed in forensic patient's pathology
Level 2	*Functional support*
Methodology	Advice plus insight-based interventions
Frequency	Weekly—monthly; can be in short bursts
Primary aim	Increase carers' capacity to reflect on and respond to the emotional needs of the forensic patient; the focus is on their role as parents or carers
Indicators of suitability	Carers see themselves as working in partnership with professionals, and able to accept support and seek a better understanding of the forensic disability patient
Level 3	*Functional change*
Methodology	Couple or family therapy
Frequency	Weekly
Primary aim	To address difficulties in the family functioning that are affecting the care of the forensic disability patient
Indicators of suitability	Carers are able to acknowledge that some of their problems lie with them and not just with the forensic disability patient
Level 4	*Psychotherapeutic*
Methodology	Individual or joint psychoanalytic psychotherapy
Frequency	At least once-weekly, long-term
Primary aim	Development of insight
Indicators of suitability	Motivated to change, psychological mindedness, ability to share or delegate primary caring roles when necessary

Figure 2. Levels of familial intervention.

and, in doing so, wish also to broaden its remit to work also with siblings of patients, whose therapeutic needs are often neglected.

Level 1 interventions are of use to those families whose experiences of the primary parental and the secondary forensic trauma have combined to reduce their capacity to think and to reflect. To focus the therapeutic spotlight on them would be too intrusive, and would, in many cases, cause them to withdraw themselves and their child from any interventions that are offered to them. The primary aim is to ensure that the therapy with the forensic disability patient is sustained. A purely educative, information-based approach allows a tacit recognition of the extreme pressures the family is under and the resultant need for specialist advice on how to manage potential overwhelming situations, while not flooding the family with a psychologically informed discourse. This level is designed to notice and respect the defence mechanisms put in place by the family, shoring up their capacity to manage situations of potential enactment. Monthly sessions are recommended, most often described as parental review meetings, which have as their stated aim the ongoing review of how the primary patient is progressing, and how the family is responding to changes in their psychological functioning.

Level 2 interventions build on the paradigm of level 1 by inserting insight-based interventions alongside information and advice, designed to allow the family to develop an emotional vocabulary with which to describe the psychological pressures of caring for someone who presents as a danger to others. Suitability for working at this level depends upon the family's capacity to form a secure alliance with the professional offering this support, and their interest in considering the emotional world of the primary patient. This level is not suitable for families who are stuck in a very regressive and defensive dynamic with service providers, unless they are somehow able to imagine the possibility that the whole world is not against them, and that there can exist others who can identify with their pain.

Level 3 retains as its focus the therapeutic needs of the primary patient, but furthers this aim through therapeutic interventions that seek to elicit change within the family unit. It is dependent upon a fairly robust family dynamic that can accommodate a level of challenge from without. This level most closely resembles family or couple therapy, occurring on a once-weekly basis, examining the dynamics of the couple or the family, specifically focusing on how those dynamics affect the primary patient. It is inevitable in many cases that this level of intervention would help individual family members to form connections between the trauma personified by the primary patient and any individual trauma they themselves have experienced. It is important that once the work reaches this level it is held and contained, rather than excavated and analysed. Such intensive individual therapeutic work lies in the province of level 4.

John and Rita fulfilled the criteria for Level 4 intervention, and, in fact, it was my conclusion that to attempt any lesser level with them could have been a misreading of their needs and capacities, and could have sabotaged the work with Maureen. I wish now to examine cases where the contra-indicators for individual or joint psychotherapy necessitated interventions at each of the preceding levels.

"Linda" and "Jerry": Level 1—educative

"Linda" and "Jerry" are struggling to deal with the increasing risk presented by "David", their nine-year-old son. He is the youngest of three boys, all of whom have autism. Jerry is a highly successful businessman, spending much of the week travelling the motorways of Britain, usually seeing his family at weekends, or, as two of the boys tend not to go to bed until near midnight, at the end of an extraordinarily long day. Linda has an internet jewellery business, although the amount of time she has to devote to it is dependent on how difficult David has been. He has a compulsion to touch other children in the genital area and has been expelled from a number of schools following complaints about his relentless pursuit of other children. He appears to have no concept of others as human beings capable of their own thoughts and feelings. His sexual enactments have a feverish, masturbatory quality to them, as if he is experiencing his victims as a part of himself. Instead of an intent to abuse, his forensic behaviour has another aim, to self-sooth, to quieten the anxieties he seems unable to put into words. His verbal language is limited. He tends to ask the same limited range of questions over and over again—often a surreal, unanswerable question, such as, "Do coconuts need to have a shave every day?" and "Will the match go out if you paint it with water?"

Linda and Jerry mirror many of David's autistic traits. Jerry struggles to think about the feelings of the children David has abused, focusing instead on his rage at their parents for "making our life hell". He desperately wants David to stop his abusive behaviour and is convinced that medication will be the solution. He has spent hours researching the internet to find a pharmaceutical answer to the dreadful question David's behaviour raises. Linda has more compassion towards David's victims, although she wishes too that their parents would "stop harassing us—we've done nothing wrong". David's behaviour has isolated them terribly, and the whole family has become removed from their community, living their lives in an autistic bubble. David's brothers are suffering too, and one of them has begun to be physically aggressive towards David, forcing their parents to remove all sharp knives from the home following a vicious attack on David by an outraged and unstoppable brother.

In assessing Linda and Jerry, I found myself almost immediately engulfed by a suspicious and rather paranoid countertransference response. I found that I lacked spontaneity in how I spoke with them, anxious about saying anything that would turn them against me. They regarded me with suspicion, particularly when, on being questioned, I revealed I did not believe that the answer to all of David's problems lay in finding the right tablet for him to take. They also grew angry when I tried to think with them about the function of their rage towards the children of David's victims. Very simple, explanatory interventions, such as, "It must be terrible to face so much anger from these people," magnified rather than contained their rage, to the point where Jerry ended up speaking, uninterrupted, for over ten minutes about "those monsters", while Linda nodded furiously, jumping in at several points with another example of the root of their problems being the actions of their neighbours. To be fair to them, David's actions had provoked much anger amongst the parents of his victims, provoking a form of vigilantism against Linda and Jerry, to the point where they seemed to be identified as the abusers as strongly as David. I was, however, concerned about his parents' failure to think about where the neighbours' anger may have stemmed from, how frightened they may have been, and how similarly Linda and Jerry would have felt had any of their sons been sexually abused. Their failure to think symbolically or to have empathy for David's victims (both the primary as much as the secondary victims) made me wary about attempting any in-depth psychotherapeutic work with them. Instead, they needed a period of supportive information and advice-based work to help them learn to think more about the situation they were in, before they might be able to move to a deeper, more reflective therapeutic level.

My primary role here was to ensure that David's psychotherapy could progress without the threat of sabotage from either parent. In order to do this, I needed to find a way of engaging with them that did not magnify their rage, nor prematurely deconstruct the massive defences they had erected against feeling more authentically the family trauma their son personified. With this level of defensive, concrete functioning, parents can be helped by an educative approach, in which the primary aim will be to help them learn about new ways of understanding their child's behaviour. Their ego strength is too weak to tolerate more explorative, psychodynamically oriented work, although as the work develops and they begin to feel more attached to the space, it should become more possible to experiment with tentative interpretations, to gradually move the focus of the sessions from a purely educative to a more integrated psycho-educative stance.

I was careful to restrict their work to once-monthly sessions. This was a struggle for both parents, as when David's therapy began his mother tended to want to bookend each session with a discussion with me about how the session had gone and, inevitably, how terrible David had been since our last session. I put in place once-monthly meetings which were divided in two: the first half examined David's therapeutic progress, while the second half examined incidents that had occurred during the month. Managing the boundaries was always a struggle, as both Linda and Jerry demanded to know exactly what was going on in David's sessions. They were particularly anxious to know what, if anything, he was saying about them, and responded badly to my attempts to remind them that confidentiality could only be broken if there were clear issues of risk and danger, if it was felt that he could be on the edge of acting out sexually. Despite this, they engaged with determination in the work. The concrete, boundaried structure of the sessions began, over time, to appeal to their rather autistic perspectives, and it began to feel as if an interesting parallel process was beginning to develop, with David's explorations of the idea of a theory of mind (Ruffman, Slade & Crowe, 2002; Proctor & Beail, 2007) echoing the awakening of his parents' interest in the thoughts and feelings of others. They had previously lacked the capacity to think about David's feelings or their own. Instead, they fixated on his actions, just as they had dwelt obsessively on their neighbours' actions instead of the feelings that underpinned them. From this, something more reflective seemed to grow, something that Jerry began to refer to as "enjoying being in class". They had both begun to joke about this new experience of being taught and its reawakening of younger parts of them that seemed to have been washed away by the onslaught of parenting at least two deeply troubled children. It was in response to this that I suggested that they may also, in fact, have much to teach—given that they were the real experts in relation to their son. Perhaps they could begin to formulate some of their own theories about why he was so drawn to perverse behaviour? Our year of looking at various theories of the aetiology of sexual enactments had equipped them to think more carefully about perversion as being a multi-causal phenomenon—one that rarely had one cause and thus rarely just one form of treatment.

Parents working at this stage of educative input may also benefit from such interventions as video interaction guidance, in which the parents are guided to reflect on video clips of successful interactions with their child (Kennedy, Landor & Todd, 2011). Through focusing purely on the positive, parents are helped to notice that such moments tend to revolve around attunement to the child's needs for attachment, thus helping them to build upon these moments, eventually embedding them in their overall interactions with their child.

"Ayesha": Level 2—functional support

"Ayesha" is the main carer for her brother "Rahul", and has been since the death of their mother ten years ago. Rahul is thirty-eight, four years older than Ayesha, and has mild intellectual disabilities. On one level, he functions well. He can read and write, and takes great pride in his appearance. He is good-looking, with a strong interest in clothes and an ever-growing collection of style magazines from which he chooses his latest look. To see him in the street is not to see someone with an obvious disability. His appearance tends, however, to mask an internal state of chaos. Since childhood he has had a compulsion to expose himself in public, usually, though not exclusively, to middle-aged women. This compulsion has caused him to be expelled from schools and colleges, and to lose the few part-time jobs he has managed to get. It seems clear that his compulsion is fuelled by anxiety, with his acting out spiking at those times when he seems overwhelmed by feelings of self-hatred. The bright, fashionable clothes he swathes himself in mask a painfully thin skin. It does not take more than an off-hand comment by a stranger on a bus to connect Rahul with barely repressed feelings of utter self-loathing. In his therapy he is working hard at articulating those feelings in the hope that the more he can use words to verbalise his ongoing sense of pain the less he will need to inflict it upon others. Humiliation is never far from his thoughts, and his compulsion to show his genitals to unknown women may be an attempt to pass on his shame to someone other than himself, and, of course, someone who is in many ways representing to him a maternal object.

Ayesha has functioned as a quasi-mother to Rahul for some time, and the contours of her life have been shaped by his support needs. He lives in semi-independent accommodation, but spends most of his weekends in the house that Ayesha shares with her partner and their four-year-old son. It is an arrangement that Ayesha both wants and resents. She holds a strong sense of responsibility towards her brother, and struggles with deep feelings of shame that he cannot live with her full-time—something she feels that her mother would have wanted her to offer. In her first meeting with me, Ayesha described herself as "mother, father, and sister" to Rahul, adding, "and a bit of a social worker, too, when there's time". She works in the IT department of a local college and has been trying to study for further qualifications, in order to progress in her career. She speaks about Rahul with a mixture of exasperation and love. "He's a worry, a really deep worry," she says, "and I don't understand what makes him do what he does. It's wrong. It's totally wrong, but I don't think he understands that. Everyone has tried so hard with him, to get him to change, to try to understand why he shouldn't do it. But he just carries on, keeping on doing it." When I explore whether there are any issues in Rahul's childhood that might explain his forensic behaviour, Ayesha shuts down, saying, repeatedly, "I don't know. I can't know." There is a quiet desperation in her eyes as she says this, and I am left with a powerful feeling that the "can't know" outweighs the "don't know." It will take much work for her to be able to think less defensively about not only Rahul's childhood, but hers too. She hints at having had a violent father, but shuts the conversation down when I try to tread too closely to this.

She comes more alive when we talk about how she should deal with the various emotional crises that Rahul brings to her home at the weekend. He is prone to extreme anxiety and bouts of depression, while also plaguing her and her partner with the need for constant reassurance that they are not going to stop inviting him to their home. She responds well when I encourage her to think about various practical ways in which she could help Rahul manage his anxiety. She is able to formulate ideas herself about ways of allowing Rahul to know he can talk more about his feelings without his world imploding. I pepper some of our conversation with tentative interpretations about the weight she carries. She tends to shrug these off. She has a practical mind, and will often try to fend off attempts by me to think with her more creatively about the sadnesses of Rahul's life, and its impact upon her, with a stock phrase: "It is what it is." I come to dread this phrase, coming as it does at those moments when I feel she is getting close to taking in something more creative, something more relational. It is often just too terrifying for her to allow herself to wonder what life would be like if *it wasn't what it was*. I come to realise that she is petrified of exploring her own history, meaning that the emphasis has to be mainly on Rahul's narrative. She is too defended to tolerate interpretations into either the aetiology of Rahul's forensic enactments or into early family history (or, indeed, the potential link between the two).

I often wonder what it must have been like to grow up in the shadow of this older brother, with all his surface sheen and beauty hiding such immoveable feelings of self-hatred. I wonder when she first began to notice that she was overtaking him intellectually, and what complex mix of satisfaction and shame that may have left her with. This is a narrative that may take years to emerge, and for now the most she can manage is to accept gentle invitations to not just attend to the practicalities of Rahul's problems, but to the intricate emotional confusions they are masking. She has the ego strength to deal with some interpretations, but her tightly constructed defences mean that they have to be diluted by solid advice and information as, without that, she could feel herself to be adrift on a sea of trauma.

The Wade family: Level 3—functional change

"Philippa" is twenty-five, and has moderate to severe intellectual disabilities. She lives with her family. She has poor verbal communication skills but has learned to use behaviours to let others know about her feelings, thoughts, and desires. She was initially referred to the clinic I worked in for risk assessment, followed by psychotherapy. Her parents worked hard to place her in a highly regarded special school when she was five, and she blossomed there, exceeding the limitations of her disability and seeming to be on the road to transcending some of the limits of her cognitive deficits—a tribute to the power of well-attuned, psychologically informed education. She was the victim of a sadistic sexual assault when she was ten. The attack was perpetrated by a gang while Philippa was on a school holiday, a seaside holiday that had been the first real break she had had without her family. Following that, she regressed, her disability becoming more pronounced, her confidence disappearing, and her previously bright demeanour replaced by a haunted, anxious depression. Her parents and twin brothers, Joe and Paul, were similarly affected by the attack. Mr and Mrs Wade withdrew her from the school, and attempted to educate her at home, giving up their jobs in the process. Joe and Paul, two years younger than Philippa, found their home turned into a mixture of school and day centre, with their bright, loving sister having turned into a dark, worried, and worrying stranger.

The family struggled on for three years until finally having to admit that they were unable to give Philippa the education she needed, and she began attending a local special school. The experiment was not a success, as Mr and Mrs Wade found Philippa's absence impossible to bear. They accompanied her to and from the school, and sought to interrogate her teachers on a daily basis about how she had been, eventually making a series of complaints against the teaching staff on the grounds of negligence. She was moved to another school and the cycle began again, continuing in various forms ever since. The battle for Philippa and against whatever setting she was in became Mr and Mrs Wade's main occupation. Their home changed from a school to a campaign headquarters, with rooms bursting with files of correspondence, letters of complaints and records of endless disputes between the Wades, local authorities, teachers, and social workers.

Things got worse when Philippa was twenty-three. She absconded from home and was found two days later in a bus shelter with a four-year-old girl she had kidnapped from a local shopping centre. She had subjected the girl to what is thought to have been a sadistic vaginal attack, although, since Philippa has never been able to talk about exactly what she did, and the girl has been similarly unable to disclose any of the details, the exact nature of the attack has remained unclear. No police action was taken, owing primarily to Philippa's intellectual disability and the girl's parents' unwillingness to press charges, but the impact on her life was catastrophic. Since that day she has remained under a form of house arrest. Her parents blame her social worker for the attack, along with the day centre that Philippa was attending at the time. They are suing the local authorities, and have enlisted the help of their MP, while also starting a charity whose aim is to campaign for higher standards of residential and day care for people with intellectual disabilities. The fight has become their life. In the meantime Philippa has regressed further, developing a compulsion to masturbate herself on average six times a day, often in the kitchen or living room.

For the Wades to allow Philippa to have a risk assessment and then to enter psychotherapy was a major achievement for them, and was made possible by a tenacious social worker who used her skills of empathy, honour, and resilience to slowly win the trust of Mr and Mrs Wade. She empathised with their rage, avoided any statements that could be heard as identifying with the authorities, and commended them on their bravery, allowing them to have a unique experience of a representative of failed authority to be accorded some level of trust. As part of Philippa's referral process, I met with Mr and Mrs Wade, and was astonished by the level of visceral rage they brought into the room. They spoke, almost uninterrupted, for over an hour about the various ways in which Philippa had been failed by services, their affect growing more agitated the longer they spoke. Eventually I was able to intervene, saying how much I sympathised and identified with what it is like to have to deal with insensitive and unresponsive systems, and how struck I was by how hard they had had to work to create a good, healthy family system themselves. They took this in, and I then asked about Joe and Paul, about their thoughts and feelings about Philippa. This question evoked more rage, as they told me how blighted their sons' lives had been, and how furious the boys were too. We were out of time, and I suggested that Joe and Paul come into the next session to meet with me so we could learn something about their perspective—something the parents readily agreed to.

I was struck on first meeting Joe and Paul by how un-twinned they seemed. Joe was clearly fuelled by the same rage as his parents, and he spoke with similar vitriol and using similar language about the failure of services to give Philippa anything of what she needed. Paul was quieter, and halfway through the session I wondered what it was he wanted to say and whether it was hard for him to speak out. He smiled and said that it was, indeed, difficult to be heard in the family, particularly when he wanted to talk about how the family was, and how much their dysfunctions may have contributed to the horrific way in which Philippa's life had turned out. This evoked a tremendous wave of anger from Mr Wade, who accused Paul of being "a turncoat" and of "letting the side down". There then followed an enactment of the family's propensity to defend through attack, with Paul seeming to personify for the rest of his family the cruel, unthinking, and abusive outside world against which the family had to constantly battle. Eventually I was able to make myself heard and I suggested that the minute the family fight amongst themselves it must feel as if nowhere is safe. The danger wasn't out there, in all the social workers, teachers, and other professionals who had failed them; it was here, inside the family unit. Perhaps, I suggested warily, this space could be one in which different thoughts and feelings could be explored safely, where the family could start to learn something new about how they functioned and how their functioning impacted upon Philippa.

The work with the Wades had in common with level 1 work the primary aim of ensuring that Philippa's therapy was not sabotaged. It would have been unsurprising if, without the building of an alliance between the family and the clinic providing the therapy, at some point they had turned against the clinic and terminated the therapy. The work had an additional aim, however: that of addressing the family's disabled way of functioning and the forensic way in which their anxiety-driven aggression threatened to magnify Philippa's difficulties. While they were not ready to work at level 4, they benefitted from a level 3 intervention that slowly enabled them to understand and better manage the rage that had been externalised for so long upon a frightening and chaotic world. They required some directive interventions to help them not only to manage their rage, but also to understand the underlying motor of their fury. At heart, their grievances stemmed from grief—the grief of having a daughter with a disability, a child that would not be cherished by the world, alongside the compounding grief of her experiences of sexual abuse, and her unconscious attempts to master that trauma through externalising it upon a child. While being helped to better manage their internal rage, to allow Paul's quiet voice to be heard amongst the clamour of their enraged voices, and to begin to move from a view of the world as a persecutory object, they were also learning how to mourn a complex and profound series of losses. While the work was structured more tightly and was more educative and directive than what we might call the "purer" therapy that John and Rita benefitted from, the Wade family did begin to internalise a gentler, more reflective way of thinking about themselves.

On first reading, it may seem surprising that Ayesha was less able than the Wades to benefit from a more psychotherapeutic approach. In assessing her needs it became clear that her defences against thinking were extremely tightly constructed, added to which she tended to buttress these defences through using intellectualisation, often discussing highly emotive issues in a dry, academic, and dispassionate way. I judged that the Wades, for all their rage and volatility, actually possessed more potential to begin to allow a different voice to be heard in their sessions, a voice they were able to introject and internalise over the course of the work.

* * *

It is clear that the category of approach used is based in part on the needs of the forensic disability patient, but also on the psychological availability of the family. Rustin (2000) emphasises the importance of assessing the fragility of the parents and their ability to work on the proposed level, while Green (2000) amplifies the need to assess the affective capacity of the parents to acknowledge that the child is not only dependent on and attached to them, but also a separate and developing individual—a key difficulty for many parents of patients with intellectual disabilities and far from confined to purely forensic cases.

Having a child with a disability inevitably tests how solid the foundations of the family are. To have a child with a disability involves a complex process of grief for the loss of the imagined baby—a process that requires an optimal mixture of good internal working models on the part of the parents, and an equivalent robust system of support and care on the part of society. It is rare that the two phenomena coexist. The path of healthy development for a child with disabilities is often compromised by unresolved mourning on the part of his parents, exacerbated by a powerful societal denial of the need to grieve. I have been struck by how many parents I have worked with over the years have transformed grief into grievance. The danger of this happening is exacerbated by genuine failings in the general provision of care for children and adults with disabilities. As has been seen in the preceding vignettes, it is rarely enough to just be a parent or a sibling of a child with disabilities. The role also requires a tenacious ability to fight services for funding and facilities, and a capacity to understand care systems that tend to be as disabled as the people they serve. There is good reason to be angry, but what I am describing is a more traumatogenic rage in which the care system becomes an irredeemably bad object, soaking up all the family's frustration, impotence, and loss. What the various levels of intervention are seeking to do in differing ways is to analyse a pathological transference process in which the system is never just the system; it is the bad object. It has come to represent whatever vindictive supreme being or universe deprived them of their longed for child in the first place. Until this can be understood it is likely that grievance becomes a perversion in and of itself, a sadomasochistic process in which true satisfaction can never be attained, where hatred keeps both hated and hater in fixed positions to each other.

The narrative of the sibling of a child with intellectual disabilities is often an unvoiced one. To have a sibling with intellectual disabilities often involves not just growing up in an atmosphere toxified by unresolved grief, it also means learning how to live with unexpressed and unmet needs. It was at a relatively late stage in their therapeutic work that both Joe and Paul began to talk about their envy of the time and care lavished upon Philippa throughout their childhood, and beyond, with Paul in particular articulating his conflicting feelings of love and hate for his sister, an ambivalence that for some time he held alone for the family before they were able to share it more equally amongst themselves. Over time the family were finally able to voice without shame the ambivalence they felt about Philippa; just as, in her own therapy, Philippa was able to voice the ambivalence she felt about them. While Ayesha was further away from this more integrated and nuanced way of thinking about the impact her brother had made upon her life, the more she was able to experiment with tentative interpretations about how hard it had been to have a life shaped so much by disability and trauma, the more hopeful I could feel that she could progress from one level to the next.

The levels of intervention suggested in this chapter should not be interpreted as being static ones, with no movement from one level to another. It should be hoped that some families are able to leave the confines of level 1 work, with its focus on educative intervention, to move on to level 2 work, with its added capacity to explore and develop moments of insight. Similarly, with sufficient work done with a family on level 3 functional change, it should be possible for one or more members of the family to engage in individual, couple, or family therapy that has as its primary aim the development of insight that is not so focused on the primary needs of the forensic patient. Whatever the level, the work is easier when the foundations are solid, and much harder when we encounter or observe couples who have fallen out of love with each other, either because love would have died regardless of forensic trauma, or because it has been atrophied by the cumulative pressure of disability. It is inevitable that there will be cases where the primary aim of the work moves from sustaining a couple or family to acknowledging that all that can actually be done is to acknowledge the death of the relationship in as compassionate and thoughtful a way as possible.

Every level of work must examine the two layers of trauma present in all these cases: the primary parental trauma and the secondary forensic trauma. Bálint's (1979) notion of the basic fault is a helpful reminder of the central role that object relations thinking has in our building of forensic disability theory. We are invariably dealing with families whose lives have been shaken and shattered by various earthquakes, most vividly the fact of their child's sexual enactments. While this is, of course, of enormous interest to us as forensic disability therapists, we have to be equally interested in the original fault line—the unmarked grave of the hoped for baby. Working within the parameters of whatever level our clients can withstand, we are symbolically constructing a tombstone to this imagined, longed for baby, allowing families to grieve their loss before they can move to a more integrated stage of being able to hold a healthy sense of ambivalence about the child that took its place. In essence, we are helping families move from a paranoid-schizoid position wherein the world is either utterly terrible or blissfully perfect, with nothing in between, to a depressive position (Klein, 1946) in which the agony of having a child with intellectual disabilities who abuses others can coexist with an awareness that this is not the totality of who they are. They remain a human being who can be loved as well as hated.

CHAPTER SEVEN

Sex as an SOS: group analytic perspectives

Like Freud before him, Foulkes, one of the founders of group analysis, viewed intellectual ability as a prerequisite for entry into a group. He specified that the candidate for group analysis should have a level of intelligence that was "not below average—preferably high" (1964, p. 44) while also privileging the "potential social value of (the) individual". Much has, thankfully, changed in the intervening decades, with group therapy being demonstrated as effective with people with intellectual disabilities for a wide range of emotional issues (Rose, West & Clifford, 2000; Stoddart, Burke & Temple, 2002; Beail, 2003), with its reach extending to patients with autism and other complex diagnoses (Ãvila & de Macedo, 2012). Group analytic approaches with forensic disability patients, while attracting less research attention than other approaches, do, however, have a growing evidence base (Xenitidis, Barnes & White, 2005) and may be seen to occupy an expanding place in the range of treatment options open. In this chapter I wish to examine not just the core treatment group itself, its content, processes, and boundaries, but also the environmental factors that need to be addressed if the group is not only to survive, but to be born in the first place.

Forensic group analysis would seem to contradict some of the edicts of group analysis as, for example, stipulated by Dies (1993), who advises against admitting into group analysis patients who have difficulties with intimacy or defences based on denial and impulsive behaviour patterns. These are just two of the key diagnostic features of forensic patients, and the resistance to using group analysis may stem from a similar source as the resistance to individual psychotherapy. I wish to examine the notion that group analysis of the type theorised by Foulkes and developed by those such as Yalom is, in fact, extremely well suited to the analysis and treatment of forensic disability patients and for certain patients may in fact be more suitable than individual treatment. Welldon (2011) claims group analytic psychotherapy to be "frequently the best form of treatment not only for severely disturbed sexual and social deviancy, but also for sexual abuse. Victims and perpetrators of incest share, by the nature of their predicament, a history of an engulfing, intense, inappropriate, distorted, physical and sexual relationship of a highly secretive type within the family situation … Group analytic therapy breaks through the patterns of self-deception, fraud, secrecy and collusion that are invariably present in these cases" (p. 126). Welldon's (1997) view is that group analysis offers qualities of containment and insight that are virtually impossible in a one-to-one situation, and she argues it has a particular suitability for both perpetrators and victims of sexual abuse. I agree with her views, having seen the power of a group to provide a mirror in which its members can gaze upon their reflected experiences of aggression and violation, a place in which the oscillation between abused and abuser can be thought about and contained.

In examining the use of group analytic approaches with forensic disability patients, I will use Pines' (2000) description of the group conductor's "therapeutic map", in which he delineated three core roles of the conductor:

i. dynamic administration—the creation of the group, locating its setting, and selecting its members
ii. boundaries—ensuring safety in the group, so that, for example, the exploration of aggressive feelings does not translate into violent actions
iii. interpretation—helping the group members understand their motivations and actions by putting meaning to their unconscious communications.

Yalom (1970) described a number of therapeutic factors, those elements he judged to be essential components of group analytic experiences:

Universality: The recognition of shared experiences and feelings among group members, serving to remove a group member's sense of isolation, validate their experiences, and raise self-esteem.

Altruism: The experience of being able to give something to another person serving to lift the member's self-esteem, and help develop more adaptive coping styles and interpersonal skills.

Instillation of hope: In a mixed group that has members at various stages of development or recovery, a patient can be inspired and encouraged by another member who has overcome the problems with which they are still struggling.

Imparting information: While not, strictly speaking, a psychotherapeutic process, it can be an empowering experience (for both sides of the transaction) for patients to learn factual information from other members.

Corrective recapitulation of the primary family experience: A form of transference specific to group psychotherapy. The therapist's interpretations can help group members gain understanding of the impact of childhood experiences on their personality.

Development of socialising techniques: The group setting provides a safe and supportive environment for members to take risks by extending their repertoire of interpersonal behaviour and improving their social skills.

Imitative behaviour: In which the patient observes and imitates the therapist and other group members as they show the capacity to share personal feelings, show concern, or support others.

Cohesiveness: In many ways the primary therapeutic factor from which all others flow, a cohesive group being one in which all members feel a sense of belonging, acceptance, and validation.

Existential factors: Learning that one has to take responsibility for one's own life and the consequences of one's decisions.

Catharsis: The experience of relief from emotional distress through the free and uninhibited expression of emotion. When patients tell their story to a supportive audience, they can obtain relief from chronic feelings of shame and guilt.

Interpersonal learning: Group members achieve a greater level of self-awareness through the process of interacting with others in the group, who give feedback on the member's behaviour and impact on others.

Self-understanding: This factor overlaps with interpersonal learning but refers to the achievement of greater levels of insight into the genesis of one's problems and the unconscious motivations that underlie one's behaviour.

Of the various formats of analytic group therapy, I suggest that the slow open model is most suitable for forensic disability patients. This format, in which the group is an ongoing process to which members are referred, staying for some time and then moving on while the group itself remains, can provide patients with a rich set of developmental experiences. Being born and delivered into a group, experiencing the helplessness of being the baby of the group family, having to make sense of the fact of a family history before one's existence, can be as new and as reparative as facing the ending of one's time in the group, processing all the learning that has taken place during one's life within the group, and mourning the ending of that time. The slow open model is particularly well suited to the many and complex differences in ability presented by any disability group. The most severely disabled member can be afforded a longer stretch of time in which to experience fully the expanse of the group, while those with milder disabilities or with a greater capacity to process and internalise the therapeutic experience may require less time. The model I am thinking of here requires a minimum two to three years involvement, regardless of the core level of disability. The group should take place at least once a week and preferably twice, in the same room and at the same time.

Foulkes' preference was for seven or eight as the ideal number of patients in a small group, as opposed to a median or large group (Foulkes, 1964). I suggest this is too large for a forensic disability group, as six is the largest number that can use the group both productively and safely. Forensic disability patients will inevitably seek to destroy the group space, to sabotage its boundaries, and to project into it a level of chaos and instability that mirrors closely the fragmented state of their internal landscapes. The image that came to my mind in trying to describe to a supervisor the experience of being in a room with six men of varying levels of disability and communication skills was that of being surrounded by six television sets, all tuned to different channels, all with the volume on full. Opinions vary as to whether one or two therapists are needed to work with the level of fragmentation that forensic disability patients can present. I have worked with and value both positions. The group will seek to split any parental couple, but will seek to do the same to a sole therapist, to project extremes of good and bad into him, to break down thinking and attack cohesion. Regardless of whether the therapist is part of a pair or not, the need for connection to an external partner is essential. Clinical supervision provides an external space in which the thoughts that are endlessly attacked inside the group can be held and processed.

Group analysis with forensic disability patients is most usefully considered in the context of Hollins and Grimer's (1988) three secrets: disability, sexuality, and mortality. As noted in Chapter One, these three areas can be viewed as overarching themes that do not guide the content of the group process, but act as a contextualising backdrop for it; the aim of group analysis, in its various forms, being lasting change brought about by non-directive free association. While the work of the group is most usefully conducted according to these group analytic parameters as articulated by, for example, Pines and Yalom, there remains, as there is in the context of individual psychotherapy with forensic disability patients, the need for ways in which psychoanalytically informed work can be contextualised and made accessible for those responsible for referring patients for treatment. The following vignette will illustrate some of the ways in which an analytic methodology may be seen to illustrate the group members' processing of the three secrets.

* * *

The group, today comprising five men, shuffles into the room. As always, there has been a pre-group group in the waiting room, with much chatter and laughter between the men and their carers, in stark contrast to the silence that they now bring into the room. "Stuart", who, along with "Ken" is one of the most severely disabled members of the group, gets out his camera phone and seems to be preparing to film the group. This elicits a volley of protest from the other group members, apart from "Patrick", a man with moderate intellectual disabilities and

Down's syndrome, who is excited at the idea of being filmed, and says he hopes it will be on YouTube, "so I can be a star!"

I suggest that Stuart may be letting us know how hard it is to be a member of the group—filming takes him out of the group and means he can feel safer, living behind the lens. Stuart says this is "mad"; he just wants to make a film, like they do in his day centre. I try again with my interpretation, only this time I add that he may be voicing the feelings of other men in the group who can also struggle with the pain of having of think about feelings. Stuart softens, and says he is now sorry for storming out of the previous week's group. He glares across at Ken. "He was driving me mad. I couldn't stand it anymore."

"David", a large, ungainly man with moderate disabilities suffered as the result of a childhood head injury growls across at Stuart, "Leave him alone. Bully! You're a bully!" Before I can make any interpretation, Ken defends against the agony of being attacked by Stuart by embarking on his usual set of questions of me: "Did I have a nice week? How is my (imagined) wife? How is my (imagined) car going?" There's mildly disparaging laughter from some of the other men, with one of them seeming to taunt both me and Ken by ridiculing the ritualised way in which Ken has made his questions into a weekly tradition, a litany that has, at some point in every group, to be reiterated.

Stuart repeats his wish to film the group. David pleads with me "Please, tell him to shut up!" I try to speak over the wave of laughter and shouting this remark elicits, and wonder about the men's mixed feelings about Ken's questions—questions I presume they also want to have answered. This quietens the group somewhat, and then Tommy asks, "What's going on with the parents' group? Why didn't they meet last week?" I try to pick up on the way in which, as ever, the parallel support group is called the parents' group, but the men are bored with hearing my curiosity about this, and instead embark on fantasising about why the parallel group had been cancelled the preceding week (due, in fact, to the group therapist being ill). I remark on how important the "parents' group" has become to them and I wonder what they imagine the group does.

David says, "They talk about how bad we are." For the first time in this session, a remark is not met with defensive laughter. Instead, the group seem to come together in a thoughtful, reflective quietness. Patrick says, "They want to know how much I talk about sex." Several of the men agree; this is, they imagine, exactly what their carers want to know as well. A silence opens up, one that I am reluctant to shut down, knowing how fleeting these moments of group reverie can be. It is broken by Ken, who says he has a note to show me from his social worker. I encourage him to share the note not just with me, but with the whole group but, as ever, Ken struggles with acknowledging that he is in a group at all, tending instead to relate to me as his individual therapist, albeit one with a very alive and active audience. The note reads, "Ken's group ends at Christmas. Ken is moving to a new day centre." Patrick says, "This is fucking crap. Ken's not leaving." Ken looks over at me, sadly, and then says, "I think I am. They said I am."

I notice that Stuart has picked up his phone, and seems about to try to film the group again. I say, "I wonder if, like all the group, you're worried about the group surviving, needing to film it while it's still alive." Stuart shakes his head, saying he just wants to film people's faces. Tommy says he doesn't want to be filmed, a thought echoed by the rest of the men. He then says, "I wish my probation officer came to the parents' group, but I only see him once a month." Instead of sympathy, this comment elicits derision, and a battle to claim the most attentive carer. The men say they see their workers every day and they are glad they do. This segues into a discussion about supervision and monitoring, with Patrick pointing out that he is accompanied by two members of staff wherever he goes, such is the fear that he will abuse children again. David claims to have four members of staff with him at all times and says that without them he would be in prison for rape. Throughout this Tommy looks increasingly dejected and I point out how the group is struggling to really hear his sadness and his sense of aloneness, replacing it with a race to be both the most dangerous and the most cared for man in the group. I add that we also seem to find it hard to stay with what Ken has brought in, the possibility of his being forced to leave the group. Patrick says, "Like my bastard dad." Stuart stands up to walk out of the room, saying, "Not that word as well. Not that word."

Tommy says, "He doesn't like the word s - e - x." To which Patrick responds, "S - o - s?", prompting much manic laughter. I leap on the slip, wondering if the men are sending me their distress signals—will I save their souls? Mark nods, and then describes how near he got during the week to raping his support worker. At first he blames her for exposing too much of her skin, something Stuart disputes, recalling an earlier session in which the men's propensity to blame their victims for the actions of their attackers was held up to the group light. "It's us as well," he says, fixing upon his face a wide smile, as if proud of remembering this insight. He is interrupted by Ken asking what happens if he wants to go to the toilet during the group, referring to the fact that those escorting him would be in their own group. Patrick says, "No one's ever gone to the toilet in middle of the group," to which Tommy declares, "I'll drink lots of water and coffee before the group!"

Patrick, who has been scratching his chest repeatedly, reveals that he is wearing a bra underneath his sweatshirt. He has talked before about cross dressing and this prompts other men to talk about their own interest in wearing women's clothes. I say that this seems to be about more than just clothes—perhaps it is about what male and female feelings are inside the men. Patrick says that he envies women, as they can have periods and understand pain. Tommy nods furiously at this (as a child his mother forced him to change her sanitary pads as part of her sexual abuse of him). We are suddenly at the end of the session, with little time left to interpret all that has been communicated, and prepare the men for their re-emergence into the outside world.

* * *

This group demonstrates Yalom's (1970) elements of group analysis in various ways. Despite the sadistic attacks erupting at various points through the group, there are also moments of altruism, such as when David seeks to defend Ken from Stuart's hatred and derision. While Ken remained seemingly deaf and blind for many months to these attempts to protect him from the derision of another, various men's continuing attempts to add salve to his wounds was eventually felt by him, but also experienced by all of the group. In protecting the most severely disabled from attack, the group was also voicing its collective need for protection and for nurturing, while taking up a more hopeful position. If they could understand their propensity to attack others within the group, they could feel more hopeful about the possibility of regulating their sexual aggression outside as well. The group's descent into a perverse form of auction as to who was the most escorted and therefore the most dangerous group member may be viewed as a worrying indicator of the men's need to form a hierarchy of abuse, to claim dominance over others. I came to view it also as the precursor to a more relational and educative process of sharing the differing aspects of not just their levels of supervision and monitoring, but also the forms of home in which they lived or the kinds of day services they used. As the group progressed, the men appeared to benefit both from imparting information to others about the circumstances of their lives, but also in taking in this information from others—to be able to think more insightfully about their place in the world by comparing it with another's. The group, much like individual psychotherapy, is a place in which learning is promoted, not simply within a didactic process but as an affective process too. As Foulkes says, "The aim of our psychotherapy is therefore liberation in the patient's inner psychic life from that which prevents him to change, from his inner blocks, a process of *unlearning* in a sense" (1975, p. 109). Learning occurs within the ahistoric context of the group; all that happens is both in the here and now and the then and there. Every group interaction contains a resonance of earlier dyadic and group interactions, making the group an echo chamber of early object relations.

Stuart functioned not just as the container of the men's ambivalence about the group, but also of their hatred of their disability. His valency to test and break boundaries was a useful one for the rest of the group, relieving them of the pressure of confronting their own boundary-breaking capabilities while affording them the pleasure of deriding what he did on their behalf. His anti-group (Nitsun, 2002) valency became something that could be used for the benefit of the group, his visceral abhorrence of Ken allowing himself to project into him all of his contempt for his own deficits and vulnerabilities. His storming out of groups was the enactment of a group wish to expel their disabilities from the room, and gradually stopped over the subsequent year as the group grew more able to claim back from him those parts of his hatred that were, in fact, theirs. Ken's litany of questions are recited for the benefit of the group as a way of voicing their ongoing curiosity about who I am and what I represent. The car they imagine me driving tended to be a sports car, a symbol of potency, a vehicle for power and agency that they could never attain for themselves, aside from their perverse enactments of abuse. Beneath their questions resided that most unspeakable of questions: what do I really think about them, their disability, and their offending? Am I repulsed by them, do I want to drive away from them as quickly as I can, would I far rather be with my wife than sitting with them and all they represent in terms of perversity and damage. The interpretation I found unable to formulate at the end of this group concerned the group's ongoing curiosity about what kind of parental object I could be for them. The bastard dad, full of hatred and contempt for them, or the maternal object who could, because of her own pain, understand their agony. Ultimately they were asking if I could bear to form a relationship with their disability, think with them about how their sexuality has been perverted by various trauma, and stay with them as we considered the meaning of their lives and their eventual deaths.

For most of the members of this group, this was their first experience of putting words to their feelings, of voicing their narrative and of having it heard and validated by others. The first six months of this group featured an opening "news round" in which all of the men were encouraged to share one positive and one negative experience from the week. While the content of what was shared invariably yielded rich symbolic material, the process of learning to speak and to be heard was as important and as transformative. Eventually, once this experience was internalised, to varying degrees, by the group, the round was able to be let go of in favour of a more naturalistic, unstructured sharing of the men's experiences and feelings since the preceding group. They were not just developing socialising techniques, they were also displaying positive imitative behaviour, having observed and internalised both from their therapist and their peers the relief to be had in verbalising that which had previously been encoded purely in silence, depression, and action. In pointing out that the way a victim of rape dresses does not remove responsibility from the rapist, Stuart articulated Yalom's "existential factors"—the acknowledgement of accountability for one's own life and one's own decisions. While it was some time before others actively joined Stuart in his understanding of this issue, the process of changing their perspective was an intensely painful (and thus authentic) process of interpersonal learning, akin to what Foulkes (1964) called "ego training in action". This is an essential aspect of a positive forensic group experience—the connection between insight, understanding of the self, and "outsight", the understanding of others. The capacity to demonstrate both areas of awareness tends to be atrophied in forensic disability patients and requires an extremely well attuned and rigorous group experience to achieve authentic transformation.

I would describe this session as being part of the beginning of a long, slow, and gradual process of the group forming a cohesive whole from which, eventually, the notions of disability, sexuality, and mortality could be processed on a meaningful level. I suggest that most of the cohesiveness on display here is fairly perverse, based as it is on who is the most dangerous abuser and conforming more to Hopper's notion of massification within traumatised and traumatising groups (Hopper, 2003b). Despite, however, the cohesion here being a false, defended variant, over time the group learned that a sense of togetherness did not necessarily have to stem from shared experiences of enacted perversion. It could flow instead from shared experiences of victimisation, of surviving derision and hatred from the non-disabled world, or from the growing experience of being able to verbalise their histories and have those histories heard and understood. The form of catharsis that became an increasing part of the fabric of the group's life allowed the men to balance their terror at unfurling their shame-ridden secrets of childhood with a strengthening sense of internal agency. At the heart of this session and, indeed, of the group's eventually long life, was a profound form of group transference, a process by which the men"s experiences of being the disabled baby, the abused child, or the abusing adult were not just put into words, they were played out and experienced in deeply unconscious ways.

The forensic disability group is thus able to make use not just of vertical transferences such as those encoded in the dyadic exchanges of individual psychotherapy, but also of the horizontal transferences flowing from group member to group member. This therapeutic democraticising of the analytic process allows for a rich synthesis of clinical issues. In working with the forensic disability group one is not working with a group of individuals. Unlike individual forensic psychotherapy, the "inner processes of the individual are internalisations of the forces operating in the group to which he belongs" (Foulkes, 1990, p. 212). One of Foulkes' analogies was that of the group as a jigsaw puzzle, whereby an individual does not make much meaning on his own but, on joining a group, can reconstruct the original jigsaw of his family, shaping and being shaped by the pieces around him. The group should thus be thought of as a matrix, a dynamic and alive set of interactions between singletons, pairs, subgroups, and the whole group.

A key issue to be considered in assessing forensic disability patients for group therapy is that of hetero- or homogeneity. It is often claimed that "mainstream" groups with specific goals, such as overcoming substance dependency or coming to terms with a cancer diagnosis, have a homogenous population with clearly stated aims and are more easily defined than psychoanalytic groups (Montgomery, 2002). Conducting a forensic disability therapy group calls into question the notion of homogeneity, given the extraordinarily wide range of disabilities, gradations of expressive and receptive communication abilities, and range of trauma suffered and perpetrated found in any group. There are too many variables to have a truly homogenous group. Even if all the members had, for example, moderate disabilities, it would be difficult to guarantee that they would all have perpetrated incest, or paedophilia, or whatever presenting symptom is chosen. Welldon (2011) advocates the heterogeneous forensic group, quoting a personal communication from Pichon-Riviere that the more heterogeneous the group the more therapeutic it becomes. The perversion, and society's hatred of it and those who have perpetrated it, becomes the homogenising factor. It is this, alongside the experience of having a disability and being hated for it, that forms the symptomatic glue that binds the group together.

It is impossible and unhelpful to try to examine a group process without considering the specific role of the group therapist. It is noteworthy that the group therapist is usually described as the conductor, implying in a Foulksian sense that the therapist is an *instrument* of the group. His role is to support the integration of the group, to note and explore transferences as they emerge, and to trace the evolution of projective identifications amongst the group and between the group and the conductor. The therapeutic style of the conductor will be linked as strongly to his personality as it is to his training and supervision, with an important balance needing to be struck between an unobtrusive stance and an overly dominating one. Too much intrusion will disable the men, cathecting them to early experiences of helplessness and impotency. Too little intrusion (an overly silent conductor) will allow the men to transform the group space into a perverse arena in which action triumphs over thought, and where aggressive attacks on those group members personifying the severest of disability and damage will be tolerated. Foulkes advised discrimination in calibration of support given, likening it to "a loan, wisely administered, helping recovery, but stimulating activity and self help on the part of the receiver, not delaying it or making him even more dependent" (Foulkes, 1948, p. 170). Important too is the capacity of the group conductor to make himself available to the group as someone with whom they can identify, a factor that has been linked to positive therapeutic outcome (Catina & Tschuschke, 1993).

The group conductor has "to live with the group, expose himself to the currents permeating it and him, try to divine the meaning of what is going on and the relevance of this meaning" (Foulkes, 1975, p. 108). This involves building what Foulkes called an "interpretive culture", assuming the mantle of process commentator from which position he can help the group notice and understand the streams of meta communication flowing beneath their words and actions. Given the propensity of forensic patients to seek to destroy (consciously or unconsciously), to invade and penetrate the body boundaries of others, and to defend against the threat of psychic annihilation through attack, a major component of the group analyst's role is the management of the group's boundaries. This involves examining the potential to attack both the inside and the outside of the forensic disability group. On the outside, this means ensuring that the group members are not known to each other and will have no social contact outside the group. On the inside, particularly with a mix of mild, moderate, and severe disability, the analyst will be required to be watchful for boundary breaking within the group and will, given the toxic and toxifying nature of sexual perversion, need to be mindful of his own boundaries being manipulated or broken by the power of the group's collective and individual needs.

It is rare to encounter a forensic disability patient who is not already part of a group, whether that is a family, other patients with disabilities, or a professional set of carers holding the responsibility for the care and safety of the individual. I have discussed the need for intense family and systemic interventions alongside the individual treatment of a forensic disability patient, and I am of a similar view that every forensic treatment group has to have a parallel group for the care systems surrounding the patient. It is in such spaces that we can ensure that those caring for the patient are not only briefed on the nature (but not the content) of the forensic work being undertaken, but also given a place in which the unconscious processes evoked in them through close engagement with disability and sexual aggression are attended to. Foulkes (1975) stresses the importance of therapeutic administration of each analytic group, a point developed by Woods (2003) in considering group analysis for adolescents who have abused. The space I am considering includes but is more than dynamic administration—it is a psychotherapeutic endeavour in and of itself.

The building and maintenance of a forensic disability group is a more profoundly complex and difficult endeavour than the creation and maintenance of individual treatment. Putting groups of offenders together has the potential to arouse a maelstrom of paralysing anxieties within institutions. At heart there is the fear of risk being multiplied exponentially the more offenders come together. A contagion anxiety can grip potential referrers, stemming not just from the fear of the multiplication of risk, but also from the deeper terror of disability becoming magnified. I am here reminded of Virginia Woolf's response (captured in her collected diaries) to seeing a group of people with disabilities in a London street: "One realised that everyone in that long line was a miserable ineffective shuffling idiotic creature, with no forehead, or no chin, and an imbecile grin, or a wild suspicious stare. It was perfectly horrible. They should certainly be killed" (Bell, 1977, p. 13). In isolation, disability can be taken as a kind of single dose. Grouped together within a mass of disabilities it threatens to catalyse visceral terror and hatred, saturating and drowning the observer. Instead of seeing a group of human beings we are seeing a mass of monsters, a cluster bomb of paralysing anxiety.

In order to examine and defuse this potentially annihilatory bomb, those providing forensic treatment groups have to create a parallel space, a location where explosive feelings can be contained and understood. A group for carers carries the potential for thought to be created within the group and taken back to the institution. It can be a frightening endeavour for its members, as organisational and individual defences are erected for self-protective reasons and to dismantle them prematurely, before something more functional has been erected in its place, evokes terror and uncertainty. I am of the opinion that such groups cannot be described as purely psychoanalytic in nature. Psychoanalytic concepts and ways of thinking carry frightening associations and resonances for many organisations working with disabilities, and to structure a carers support group with too rigidly analytic a frame would repel many potential members. A more structured package with analytic thinking as an implicit rather than explicit aim is far more likely to achieve its primary aims of helping to maintain the work of the primary treatment group.

The parallel group model I propose is designed to mirror and echo many aspects of the main treatment group, particularly in its use of Hollins and Grimer's (1988) notion of the three secrets of disability therapy. Just as disability, sexuality, and mortality are threaded throughout the fabric of the treatment group, they are used, in a somewhat more overt way, in the structuring of the parallel group, providing its members with a sense of structure, an important component of the psychoeducative approach. The group should be formulated as an educative experience, delivered within a psychotherapeutic context. A modular approach to the group is advised, with each of the three secrets being used as a catalyst for more detailed examinations of key forensic issues. Thus, under the *disability* umbrella, seminars can be conducted on issues such as diagnostic features of disability, aspects of autistic functioning, working with variances between expressive and receptive communication, and developmental perspectives. Under *sexuality* the group will be helped to examine such areas as risk assessment, the aetiology of sexual offending, managing risk in the community, and the impact of sexual abuse upon victims. Finally, under *mortality* the group will be working with the impact of loss, dealing with major life events, separation and attachment, psychotherapeutic approaches, and the development of empathy.

As with the level of intervention used alongside individual psychotherapy (see Chapter Six), the level and depth of the intervention needs to be calibrated according to the emotional capacities of the group members. As with the treatment group, the parallel group works to a slow open model, with carers attending for at least as long as their client does. The membership of the group can be larger than that of the treatment group, as more than one carer may attend the group. The sessions should be structured according to two levels: training input and process work. The training input involves a seminar in which material on the chosen subject is discussed, reading material is shared, and a work plenary discussion is facilitated. The process part of the group is a less structured, and equally tightly contained experience in which the group members are encouraged to reflect on the emotional impact of the material they have examined. While this should be linked as far as possible with the content of the first part of the group, it should also have the capacity to deviate, and to allow the group to free associate together, exploring whatever emerges from the material, or whatever emergencies, dilemmas, or catastrophes are occurring outside the group. Given the myriad pressures placed on the shoulders of those working with forensic disability patients in the community, it is to be expected that the group will become a place to which its members can bring their various feelings of despondency, fear, and anxiety about the work they do, the setting in which it happens, and their relationship to both.

* * *

In this vignette, the first half of the carers' group has been spent examining various approaches to risk assessment in the community.

The material presented has elicited a mixture of engagement and silence from the group. The group therapist notes that they are halfway through the session, marking the point at which they move from the training material to a wider, less structured space to which people could bring their thoughts and feelings about the material discussed. There is a long silence and the therapist notes how unusual it is to have such a silence, although she had noticed a contrast between those group members who had felt able to say much and those who had stayed quiet during the first half of the group. "Toni", whose working hours are spent shadowing her client to ensure he is never in a position where he might abuse a child in the community, says, "It made me think about how much work this is. How much time and money we spend making these men safe. But what about the other people in the place where I work? Who's worrying about them? Who's running courses on how to keep them safe? It's not fair. These men soak up so much attention, so many resources." "Jo", one of those who had hitherto remained quiet, said that she had found the material challenging, as it highlighted how few risk assessment procedures were in place at her work setting, a group home for men and women with intellectual disabilities. "Barbara", who works in a separate unit, concurs with this, saying she had found it hard to break through what had seemed to her a rather "gung ho" discussion about assessing danger. She had found it difficult to relate to the methodologies discussed, given how lacking her unit was in any kind of policy and procedure, not just in the area of sexual risk, but more generally. "It's like you were talking a different language," she says, a note of rage in her usually placid voice. "Ben", one of those who had spoken much in the discussion, said that he was alarmed to hear about settings that weren't assessing risk, although his own setting, a medium secure unit, was far from perfect. This elicited some agreement from the "subgroup" who had engaged in the discussion, with most of them saying that having risk assessment procedures didn't shield them from the terror of what might happen if someone did abuse someone in the unit or in the community.

"Gazali" says how angry she is about her workplace; they have no real policies and procedures, apart from locking up clients when it is judged they might be at risk of offending. "They don't get it because they don't want to get it," she says, her voice trembling with emotion. "They're only interested in the profit, and nothing about human beings!" Gazali's emotion seems to detonate a wave of explosive rage among the group, many of whom rail against their organisation, with Vicki shouting, "And none of them come here. It's all us workers who come to this group—no managers! They couldn't care less."

The therapist comments on the rage that has been ignited by this issue, and says how unsurprising it is that there is so much anger about such appalling organisational failings. Perhaps, however, the rage is easier to stay with than what lies underneath it—the fear, the terror of something sexually abusive happening, or, indeed, of themselves being abused by the men they are paid to care for. After a few moments of silence, Jo says that she often lies awake at night, dreading the next day at work, wondering if something awful might happen to her. "Phil", who supports one of the most dangerous of the treatment group members, says how sorry he is to hear that, and how he tends not to want to dwell on feelings of fear. He just wants "to get on with it, and not worry about it"; he is "not paid to worry". The therapist wonders aloud about what Phil has just voiced for the whole group. The desire to not worry, alongside the knowledge that the men they are supporting embody the most extreme of worries—the capacity to sexually abuse.

"Liz", who has until now been silent, says, "I sometimes hate my job." There is a silence. It stretches on for some minutes until eventually the therapist suggests, "Perhaps it's not just the job you hate. How hard it must be to not hate the men you're paid to care for, too." As the group nears its close, a couple of the group members say what a relief it is to be able to talk about hating their client without fearing being seen as unprofessional or, indeed, abusive. "I've never dared say how much I hate him," says Gazali. "We don't talk about that; it's too unprofessional. My boss would wonder if I'm not up to the job. And I can't afford to lose this job." The therapist closes the group by making a connection between the group's collective hatred of the men and the maternal and paternal hatred and rejection the men had faced in their early years. Perhaps, unlike those parents, this group might find it possible to hold a healthy sense of ambivalence wherein the hatred for the men can coexist with and be understood in the context of other feelings: love, concern, boredom, frustration, hope, and hopelessness. The group, the therapist suggests, is often in the position of a depleted mother, burdened with a baby that threatens to suck her dry, leaving her other children as starving and depleted as she. The group is reluctant to leave the room, and the therapist notes this, stressing how hard they have worked today and how hard it can be to reach a position of deeper understanding, prior to having to re-enter a world that is often so devoid of such depth of thinking.

* * *

The group articulates a common thread found in parallel work with carers of forensic disability patients: a hatred of both what they do to their victims and what they do to their carers. The expression of rage at the fate of those other clients overshadowed by the needs of the forensic patient may be heard on two levels. The conscious and understandable frustration at the shrinking of time and attention paid to those patients whose depression, self-harming or low self-esteem do not have the urgent noise of sexual perversion, alongside the less conscious outrage about how even less attention is paid to the impact of working so closely and so intimately with those who personify sexual danger. "What", the group seems to be crying, "about us?" The group offers polarised views of how best to deal with this question. They can either lie awake at night, saturated by fear, or they can put their blinkers on, paying little attention to their terror and "get on with it". The expressions of hatred for their jobs or of their organisations are real, but also metaphors for their hatred of the men for whom they are paid to care. This group is on the cusp of working more meaningfully on an issue that lies at the heart of all work with disability: ambivalence.

Attitudes towards disabilities are often reduced into polarised notions of hatred or fear, with little time taken, particularly within institutions, to consider a more nuanced concept of ambivalence (Söder, 1990). In his treatise on the need for the law to adopt a more nuanced view of victims and perpetrators of crime with disabilities Muller (2011) notes the legal system's reluctance to consider this ambivalence, a reluctance stemming from a repression of one view, love or hate, in favour of another. This repression colours most interactions, legal or otherwise, with people with disabilities, and presents a particularly powerful challenge to the parallel group. As with the treatment group, the potential for destructive splitting processes is present, with the host organisations being the receptacle of much of the group's projected rage. The therapist has to tread a fine line between acknowledging and validating the group's rage at the organisation, and taking up the more painful task of considering their own internal organisations. It would be too simplistic for this group to defend against the agony of working with sexually abusive men by continually projecting their rage into their employers. For the therapist to in any way encourage this would represent a failure of the group capacity to consider its internal processes. The hated, flawed organisation is, of course, flawed and deserving of hatred. It is also a receptacle for the group's disavowed feelings of self-hatred, and its sense of failed dependency. Much like the men in the core treatment group, this group is voicing its hunger for a solid, good enough parental figure who can contain their fears, anxieties, and helplessness.

This group can be seen as a sibling, a child, and a parent of the main treatment group. The two groups have shared parentage, being born of a desire to apply psychoanalytic understanding to acts of abuse and abusing. The carers' group lives alongside the treatment group, growing and developing at a rate that is at times quicker, at times slower. Sometimes the treatment group races ahead of the carers' group in its understanding of its pathologies, while at other times the carers' group makes swifter and deeper inroads into understanding their clients' difficulties with empathy or their struggles with viewing others as anything but sexual objects. The two groups should be viewed as interdependent, with the survival of each being contingent on the other. I have come to the view that to run a treatment group for forensic disability patients without providing an equivalent group space for their carers is a doomed enterprise, with the lack of calibration between the two groups resulting in any growth of insight in the treatment group not being matched by an equivalent growth within their host organisation.

* * *

"Jiang", a man with moderate intellectual disabilities joined a slow open group that I supervised. He had a long history of sexual assaults against children, and had been through a number of CBT and offence-focused groups before being referred to this one. His defences against trauma seemed watertight. His handicapped smile disarmed most of those who encountered him, and he thrived on being thought of as happy, jolly, full of laughs. This veneer of affability and childlike joviality was also a key factor in his abuse of children, enabling him to charm children into relating to him as a peer with whom they could experiment and be experimented upon, rather than an adult intent on subjecting them to acts of sexual violation. He had just moved into a new group home, and various difficulties between the organisation running the home and the social worker overseeing his case meant that, for his first six months in the group, no member of staff attended the parallel group. He made good progress within those months, and gained much from the experience of learning that his own experiences of childhood deprivation, neglect, and abuse were mirrored and echoed by many of his fellow group members. He was not alone. Jiang had lived most of his life as a singleton, his disability, ethnicity, and forensic compulsions marking him out as someone who could rarely, if ever, feel a part of humanity. As he began to work with the group on issues of disability, sexuality, and mortality, he began to access feelings of sadness. The defences he had constructed to protect himself from the agony of feeling began to diminish. He returned from the group to his home in a depressed mood. Gone was the mask of laughter and fun he had worn, to be replaced by a flat, affectless emptiness that caused those caring for him to wonder whether the group was causing more damage than treatment.

His team recruited a local counsellor to help Jiang deal with his increasing sadness and isolation from his peers, and, within weeks of this starting, decided to remove him from the group, a decision based on a fear that the group was making him worse. This came as a tremendous shock to Jiang and to the group, for whom the implication of someone vanishing suddenly from their midst evoked their own terrors of ejection, abandonment, and being rendered invisible. Jiang himself began to self-harm some weeks after his final session in the group, his rage at those who had pulled him from the group breast just as he was beginning to trust in its capacity to feed and nourish him having to be turned against himself. His eviction from the group was a catastrophic enactment of an anxiety that had no home. Other men in the group had been through similar periods of sadness, while others seemed more drawn to exhibiting their rage, frustration, and self-hatred through a growth in anxiety-driven aggression. Both enactments may be understood as a positive and necessary dismantling of outmoded defences, the "getting worse before getting better" process familiar to most recipients of in-depth psychotherapy. The lack of a container for Jiang's team in which they could voice their anxieties about his growing melancholia resulted in a magnification of their fears that he was unravelling. It was interesting to note that, while he was losing his place in the group, the parallel carers' group were working on the therapeutic concept of the "depressive position" (Klein, 1935)—lessons that may have been extremely useful to Jiang's team.

The absence of a secondary therapeutic space for the support network of a forensic disability patient weakens the primary source of treatment, tending, as in Jiang's case, to result in the enactment of aggressive attacks upon the treatment. At times these may be conscious, as in the case of Jiang's team, a clearly stated disbelief in the efficacy of the group. At other times ambivalence about the group may be enacted less consciously, through the group appointment being "forgotten" to be handed over from one team to another, the scheduling of other appointments prior to or immediately after the group, or the over-medicating of patients on the group day, ostensibly prompted by shows of anxiety, aggression, or depression, but unconsciously designed to limit the patient's capacity to use his group treatment. All of these enactments can best be worked with in the context of the parallel group, as it is here they can be held up to the light and understood as an enactment of organisational anxieties.

Group therapy for forensic disability patients requires an adherence to Pines' (2000) "therapeutic map", in which careful attention is paid to the needs of dynamic administration, boundary management, and interpretation. The slow open model is best suited for this patient population, affording them a space that is customised to their individual needs, levels of disability, and psychological mindedness, and that can facilitate a developmental journey through their metaphorical birth, life, and death inside the group. A maximum of six patients is the optimum number for the group, in order to afford its members sufficient time and space to explore Yalom's (1970) core elements of group analytic processing. The viability of the group is dependent on the maintenance of a parallel support group for the men's carers. Without this life support system being put in place, the group baby is unlikely to survive much beyond birth. Both groups are guided by the overarching themes of Hollins and Grimer's (1988) model of the three secrets of disability, as much as by the need for ambivalence about all three states to be examined, analysed, and processed. As has been demonstrated by this chapter's material, group analysis with forensic disability patients holds many challenges both for those in the groups as well as those conducting them. Part of its power, however, lies in its capacity to work with the key clinical issue of ambivalence in a horizontal, democratised way, whereby therapeutic insight is not simply handed down from parental substitute to quasi-child. It is transmitted amongst the men, conferring in this process a heightened ability to consider others not simply as empty objects, devoid of humanity and feeling, but as reflections of oneself, allowing a reciprocal process in which the ability to relate and to be related to can be developed.

CHAPTER EIGHT

The disabled organisation: on supervision and consultation

The forensic disability patient and therapist are a couple surrounded by and potentially shaped by a host of external influences. Psychosocial factors, the criminal justice system, the needs of victims, the workings of institutions, and the presence of families are all part of the fabric against which the therapy itself is constructed. The intensity of forensic disability therapy makes it impossible for any psychotherapist on their own to track and manage the various voices straining to be heard alongside that of the patient. Supervision is designed to relieve the therapist of this additional pressure, providing a creative space in which the dyadic interactions can be considered alongside the systemic backdrop of the case. In this chapter I wish to examine two different but related areas of supervision: individual work with the forensic disability therapist and consultative work with institutions. Both endeavours have innumerable aims, but I suggest that the overarching point of both lies in the area of boundary management. Sexual abuse is the culmination of a multitude of boundary attacks, encompassing both the psychic—the intrusion into a victim's mind—and the bodily. The forensic patient lacks a clear enough sense of boundary, both their own and their victim's, and carries within them the impossibility of knowing where they end and another begins.

To abuse another is to assume a right to their mind and to their body, and is a disavowal and a denial of the boundary that exists to give us a sense of interpersonal and relational integrity.

In positing boundary management as one of the core aims of the supervision of forensic disability therapy, I do not wish to create an artificial distinction between therapeutic work with perpetrators and victims. The propensity for some therapists to assume that a lack of boundary in their work with victims is not as potentially harmful as a lack of boundary in working with perpetrators ignores the catastrophic impact for both when the absence of boundary first experienced in the sexual crime becomes enacted once more within the therapy. It also colludes with the fantasy that there is ever since a thing as just a victim and just a perpetrator. The experience of having a psychotherapist who does not hold a strong enough awareness of the sanctity of the boundary is both consciously alluring and unconsciously terrifying for the patient. The blurring of boundaries tends to start in small, incremental ways: time added onto a session, words of comfort given too easily in the place of thought and reflection, contact being offered between sessions, and so on. Supervision has to be a place in which the meaning of such changes to the analytic frame can be thought about in the context of what Langs (1994) would call frame deviancy—an enactment of pathologies contained within the clinical material. This approach ensures not just that the unconscious meaning of any attacks on the therapeutic frame can be analysed in the service of understanding the patient's internal landscape, but also that the risk of the therapist being drawn into an incremental process of collusion with the patient's pathologies can be guarded against. The therapist who eventually sexually abuses a patient follows a remarkably predictable "natural history" of progressive boundary violations (Simon, 1999). The aetiology of therapeutic boundary violations stem from a complex interplay of pathologies of both therapist and patient, with the likelihood of gross violations stemming largely from the absence of an effective supervisory container in which to monitor the stability of the analytic frame (Gabbard & Lester, 2008).

Supervision is not just a form of protection for the individual clinician in their encounters with profoundly disturbing clinical material and all the associations with seduction, arousal, excitement, and disgust that forensic material holds. Institutions and organisations are equally vulnerable to the toxic nature of forensic material, and as susceptible to a spectrum of boundary blurring and breaking as the individual. Just as the individual psychotherapist who avoids showing their clinical work to a supervisor magnifies the risk of boundary breaking in their work, the organisation that does not allow representatives of the outside world in to observe and help think about their working practices is continually placing itself in a position of extreme vulnerability. That this vulnerability mirrors that which pervades the internal working models of their clients is beyond coincidence and adds an additional function to the role of external consultant. The organisation requires a mirror into which it can gaze, to help it work out how many of its practices, attitudes, and cultures have been and are being formed by that which is projected into it by the collective disability it seeks to house. In order to examine some ways in which a supervisory or consultative lens can help clarify and define the unconscious forces at work within both individual forensic disability therapy and the institutions in which forensic disability patients are housed, I wish to use an anonymised example of the supervision of a psychotherapist struggling to retain a sense of professional and personal integrity in the face of murderous attacks upon her work.

* * *

"Lis" settles into her chair, gathering her notes and explaining how nervous she feels about discussing her work in supervision. Before discussing the background to the patient she is working with I ask her to tell me about the setting in which she works. Her eyes water, and she explains she is a psychologist in a day centre, a tremendously stressful place in which to work. She alludes to a lack of support from her superiors, and also describes an unfeasibly large caseload, which has left her with little time to think within the workplace, and little space to recover at home, invaded as it has been by the various notes and reports she has not had the time to complete during the week. Her patient is "Peter", a thirty-five-year-old man with moderate disabilities. She has been working with him for eight months, mostly without supervision, and has finally been forced to acknowledge how alone she has felt because of this lack of a space in which to think about him with another (her employers have refused to fund her supervision, so she is paying for it herself). She sees Peter for once-weekly sessions, the work initially being requested by the psychiatrist involved in his care. Peter has a history of sexually abusing both men and women. His victims tend to have intellectual disabilities, and numerous residential and day care placements have collapsed because of the risk he presents to his peers. He has been assessed as presenting a medium to high risk of reoffending, and this is the first time a psychotherapeutic approach has been attempted with him.

Peter presented initially in his sessions with poor eye contact and tremendous problems in putting any feelings into words. For the first few months Lis felt consumed by a powerful sense of boredom when in the room with him. She worried she would fall asleep in sessions, so great was the mindlessness being evacuated into her. Peter, on the other hand, appeared intrigued by Lis, bombarding her with questions about her life outside of the day centre, the husband and children he imagined her having, and the holidays he thought of her enjoying. He grew angry when she tried to interpret his need to put the spotlight from him to her, and said that she was "like all the others", wanting to know all about him but never allowing him to know anything about them. Her ability to acknowledge this rage, to not diminish its importance and to seek to think about how much better it was for him to voice his anger rather than ignore it or act it out seemed to allow Peter to turn a corner in his work. He began to show more interest in the art materials available in Lis's room, helped in this by Lis's interest in his interest. And so he embarked on a series of drawings depicting key relationships in his life: his parents, his siblings, and the various key workers he had let himself grow attached to over his years in institutions. Despite the childlike scrawl of the drawings, a narrative emerged that said much about Peter's sense of himself as being fundamentally different and less than those he loved. The depictions of his parents and his siblings were so much more fully formed than the scrawny, tiny pictures of himself that he inserted into the background of each picture.

It was at this point in the treatment that Lis was asked to report on her work with Peter to the Clinical Director of her institution. Her first attempt at a report was rejected as being too vague, and a demand was made for more specific details of what was happening within the sessions. While Lis struggled with the ethical implications of this, Peter's attendance began to falter. The staff reported difficulties with bringing him to the session, and it was decided that the work with her should come to a close. Lis struggled to contain her rage and sorrow at this decision as she describes continuing to meet Peter in the corridors of the centre, and his confusion as to what has caused this annulment of their work. She stated how cynical she now felt about the possibility of ever conducting psychotherapy within this kind of institution and recalled some of her colleagues voicing their antagonism to the concept of providing a sex offender with the "luxury" of psychotherapy. She ended by saying that she received a call that morning that Peter had assaulted a woman in the centre and further questions were now being asked of her work with him. Lis has been asked to compile a "retrospective risk assessment", ostensibly as an attempt to ascertain whether her sessions with Peter had escalated his risk of offending.

* * *

Supervision of forensic psychotherapy requires close attunement to systemic issues (Lloyd-Owen, 1997), an attunement that becomes even more important when the forensic patient has a disability. As has been demonstrated in previous chapters, forensic disability therapy is never a dyadic process. It is a triadic exchange, requiring of the forensic disability therapist a capacity to be mindful of the vertices and angles of the triangular square: the patient, therapist, and the other, most usually the referral agent. Supervision of forensic disability therapy must hold a balance between analysis of the direct clinical material itself—the contents of the therapy session—and what might be thought of as *collateral* material—the actions and impact of the referral agent. This case demonstrates how terribly cluttered the analytic space can be—particularly when it is conducted both within an institution and by a clinician perceived as being an institutional representative—and how the impact of the referral agent can be as powerfully felt as those of the primary patient. Acting out is rarely confined to the forensic patient. All who come into contact with him, including the psychotherapist, are vulnerable to enactments of thoughtlessness, fear, and aggression. In my work with Lis I deliberately chose the language of "murder", of "assault" and of "killing off" to describe the premature ending of the therapy in an attempt to think together about the ways in which the murder weapon had more than one set of fingerprints on it. The work was not killed off just by the clinical director or just by the staff team. Lis's own lack of thought about the feelings of the team may have contributed to the therapy's loss of life.

One of the most potent causes of aggression towards the concept of forensic disability therapy is envy. Lis's colleagues' notion of Peter's psychotherapy being a luxury articulates a deeply seated and understandable drive for vengeance. Our polarised notions of good victims and bad abusers are tested by the concept of replacing punishment with treatment. The desire to enact our hatred of abuse through retribution often emerges in institutions in the form of righteous concern both for the victims of abuse who receive little or no therapy, and the indirect victims of, in this case, Peter's offences—those other men and women with intellectual disabilities who are starved of time with staff because so much of that time is devoted to the monitoring and supervision of this dangerous and unpredictable man. I suggest that the actual cause of this punitive wish to deny therapeutic treatments to offenders stems more from a personal and individualised envy. Those staff working at the front line of Peter's enactments tend to be far less well paid or resourced than those responsible for his psychological care. In this trench warfare the care staff are the lowly privates, doling out medication, assisting in the intimate care of their clients, battling against the tedium and frustration of slow, repetitive minds housed in slow, ungainly bodies. The generals of this war, the clinical directors, psychiatrists and psychotherapists of Peter's narrative, are perceived as being far from the front line, easily identified as holding a level of power that is in inverse proportion to the direct work they do. The only weapons the privates have are projections, whereby the generals can become as hated and denigrated as the patient himself.

I know from the very early days of my career as one of the privates, working as a care assistant in homes and day centres for people with intellectual disabilities, how easy it can be to resent any time and money spent on those who have perpetrated abuse, and how much easier it is to express that resentment on behalf of other clients than on behalf of oneself. The lack of a constructive, rather than destructive, space for Peter's staff to express their envy of precious and finite therapeutic resources being expended on him led indirectly to the premature killing off of his treatment. They could have been helped to understand the aetiology of their envy in meaning-making ways rather than enacting it through unconscious sabotaging of his sessions. Their unconscious desire was to wrestle from Peter the "luxury" of being listened to. Their, and Peter's, tragedy was that, deprived of the luxury of putting words to feelings, he had to resort to replacing words with perverse actions. If Lis had in the early stages of constructing the container for her work with Peter considered more thoughtfully the inevitability of the staff team and the clinical director enacting their ambivalence of the therapy through a sabotaging of it, just at that moment when something more hopeful was beginning to develop, perhaps her work could have been allowed to continue.

Forensic psychotherapy with patients without disabilities is often subject to immense pressures from the outside world, most usually in the form of demands for information concerning risk and danger from agencies such as the probation service or the police. This weight is magnified exponentially when the patient has a disability, making the creation and maintenance of boundaries around the clinical work an extremely problematic issue. Services for people with intellectual disabilities can often enact an unconscious and powerful propensity to dehumanise their clients, regarding them as possessing less value than people without disabilities and requiring less care in relation to their human rights. The lives of patients with disabilities tend to be open books. It is worryingly normal for intimate and private information about patients with disabilities to be shared amongst professionals without any regard being paid to the concept of confidentiality. In order to facilitate a clinical process by which clients can internalise an authentic sense of their therapy being a private and untrespassed space in which all thoughts and feelings can be uttered without fear of consequence, a boundary has to exist between the therapy and the other domains of the client's life.

This presents a complex challenge to services, particularly those already traumatised by the pressure of caring for patients whose thoughts and actions place them at risk of committing acts of sexual abuse. Even when it is the institution itself that has referred the forensic disability patient to psychotherapy, it is difficult for it to sign up to the notion of clinical confidentiality, as it contradicts the common culture of limited or no confidentiality that pervades most dealings with patients with disabilities. The boundaries that contain psychotherapeutic work tend to be fundamentally different from those that govern institutional life and, as such, present an enormous challenge to both domains. There is an immense curiosity about what is going on between therapist and patient. While the shroud of confidentiality tends to be fairly threadbare generally in the lives of people with disabilities, the suspicion or the knowledge that someone has perpetrated acts of sexual abuse render it completely invisible. There are, of course, varying levels of curiosity that are held by those outside of the therapeutic dyad. Some of it is important and necessary—some knowledge of the broad themes being examined may be invaluable to a staff team uncertain about how to tailor their psychological responses to their client. Some curiosity may be prurient and intrusive, while also symptomatic of the inevitable anxiety aroused by the possibility of sexual attacks, and emblematic of the weight of responsibility felt by members of the patient's support network. Forensic disability therapists will find themselves asked to comment on such areas of their patient's life as the content of their masturbatory fantasies, the objects of their sexual desires, or the progress of their recollections of their histories of sexual abuse. They may also find themselves facing confusion and antagonism when they attempt to draw a clear therapeutic boundary around their work.

The protective membrane surrounding the therapeutic work can be worn thin by requests that take on the quality of aggressive attacks. Supervision must equip the supervisee with a clear sense of how permeable or impermeable the skin surrounding the therapeutic work will need to be. There is a risk of the protective layer being either too rigid (antagonising those referral agents on whom the sustenance of the work depends) or too loose (allowing members of the patient's support network to know too much about the treatment, leaving the patient feeling as if therapy is, like so many other parts of their life, an open book). Regulating this requires an understanding of the dynamics of the institution, in order to understand more completely whether the nature of the intrusion is benign, malign, or a mixture of both. Psychotherapy for people with intellectual disabilities is often denigrated by institutions and their representatives, whose disdain for therapy may be underpinned by a deep-seated envy of the patient for getting what they do not—a safe, contained space in which to think, feel, and express.

To ascertain the ratio of malign/benign intrusiveness, an ecological perspective should be taken in which all elements of the institutional matrix can be seen to impact profoundly on each other. At all times this should be linked back to and connected with the psychodynamics of the patient's therapy, and the therapist's countertransference. Taking as one example Lis's initial countertransference of boredom when with Peter, supervision had to act as a kind of psychological GMS, mapping the various locations of boredom inside and outside the patient's analytic dyadic work in order to make sense of the unconscious functions of this boredom. The boredom felt by the therapist may not just be a distillation of the patient's boredom with his own atrophied mind; it may capture the boredom felt by the patient's institution. One must also be alert, as a supervisor, to one's own feelings of tedium. The supervisor, in experiencing something of the boredom away from the intensity of the analytic encounter, may be more alive than the therapist to the organisation's inert lack of vitality and its frustration with the dead minds it has to house. Gallego (2006) describes life in an institution for people with disabilities as an ongoing experience of seasons blending into each other, the seeing of the same faces and the hearing of the same conversations—everything having a deadening, monotonous regularity. Villa (2013) describes the risk of workers' curiosity and surprise about those they work with being flattened by the bureaucratisation of activities and routines, with routine providing both boredom and reassurance. Villa locates this phenomenon particularly in working with patients with severe disabilities, whereby the lifelessness exhibited by the patients becomes introjected by their workers, leading to "an unrestrained weariness … a frustration that despises hope" (p. 137).

Supervision has to be alive to the dangers of forensic disability therapists defending against the trauma of disability by becoming "super-able". This over-compensatory defence can involve therapists taking on too many cases, promising unrealistic change to patients and to referrers, and generally avoiding the messy, frustrating, and unresolved reality of life as a forensic disability patient. The supervisor has to consider with their supervisee the risk of defences becoming concretised, and fears generated by such close contact with the twin traumata of disability and sexual aggression resulting in a form of narcissistic grandiosity—the therapist who can never say "no". Few are immune from the seduction of this form of narcissism, of course, and the supervisor must monitor their own susceptibility to contamination. Unless monitored carefully supervision sessions can mirror too closely the over-compensatory structure of treatment sessions, with both spaces becoming too full, and both supervisor and therapist echoing the patient's need to kill thought by action. Ogden (2005) describes a form of "guided dreaming" in which the supervisor provides a frame that ensures the supervisee's freedom to think and dream and be alive to what is occurring in the analytic and the supervisory relationship, as well as in the interplay between the two. He is also interested in supervision providing both supervisor and supervisee with permission to have "time to waste", enabling a type of freely associative thinking that enhances the range and depth of what can be learned from the supervisory experience.

In analysing her responses to the killing off of her work with her patient, Lis sometimes seemed to merge with Peter, voicing, on both her own and his behalf, intense feelings of powerlessness, fear, and anxiety. All power seemed to have been surrendered to the institution, with Lis presenting with a level of disability and lack of agency that seemed, on a purely emotional level, to be equivalent to Peter's. The danger of over-identification with disability is high, particularly when working with forensic disability patients, with supervision needing to function as a form of psychic barometer with which to guard against the attendant danger of overcompensation and burn out. Supervision shares with forensic psychotherapy the need to hold an archaeological perspective on all contemporaneous manifestations of trauma, and a certain valency on Lis's behalf to defensive, compensatory overwork may be seen in her over-filled workload. She had failed to hold a clear boundary, taking on every case referred to her and acting as a kind of über-therapist, in an unconscious attempt to defend against the lack of ability experienced by her clients. It is far easier to disavow lack, damage, and disability through the manic defence of overwork than it is to sit with the disability, to allow the fundamental lack embedded in every forensic disability patient to be fully held in mind.

This dynamic is not unique to individual and dyadic work. Menzies Lyth (1960) identified the many kinds of social structures created by institutions as a form of defence, to avoid experiences of anxiety, guilt, doubt, and uncertainty. One finding from my work with Lis was that the dynamics of her institution appeared too fragmented to allow forensic disability therapy to occur without the ongoing threat of sabotage and annihilation. This particular institution brought to mind Kernberg's (1993) concept of "paranoiagenesis"—his attempt to describe those organisations, mostly structurally unsound ones, where paranoid-like states prevail, particularly when their stated tasks cannot be accomplished. The level of scapegoating of Lis and of psychotherapy can be understood as a group defence against unacceptable emotions (Scheidlinger, 1982), stemming from an organisational confusion, common in many disability organisations, about what its primary tasks are. Did it exist to house and care for people with disabilities? Was its primary duty to Peter's victims, to Peter himself, or to those staff tasked with caring for and protecting both abuser and abused? Was the primary role of therapy insight-building, empathy development or risk management? The failure of the institution to think about any of these questions without becoming mired in its own confusion meant that thought became impossible, to be replaced by catastrophic action—on the part of the institution, to kill off the therapy; on the part of Peter, to assault a woman. This was a case that required not just individual supervision of the therapy, but the provision of organisational consultancy.

Hopper (2012) notes that consultations to traumatised organisations are always disturbing to the consultant. This is undoubtedly the case in consulting to organisations working primarily with disability and requires of the consultant an awareness of the propensity of organisations to embody the symptomology of those they work with, as well as an awareness of the particular political history of disability institutions. The culture of privatisation and individualisation kick-started in the UK from 1979 onwards introduced a seismic shift in the nature of relationships between institutions and the community. Long (2012) links these societal shifts to what various writers have termed "failed dependency" (Miller, 1993; Hopper, 2003b)—a societal loss of faith in public institutions and private corporations. This is particularly apposite to institutions working with people with intellectual disabilities, so many of which have been created with the primary aim of generating profit, relegating to secondary and tertiary roles the well-being of their clients and their workers. The threat of annihilation is particularly prevalent in institutions working with patients with disabilities. As funding for services for the disabled has been systematically slashed, institutions have become paralysed with terror, where the fear of redundancy and loss of income has replaced the primary tasks of care, nurturing, and support.

All of these factors can result in a form of disabled organisation in which clear thinking and communication can be subverted through the terrible price paid through the struggle to survive. Institutions can identify too closely with the disabled baby, occupying a liminal, precarious place in the world. The baby and the institution carry shame on behalf of mother, father, and society. They are starved of resources by a society that would rather they died, as they represent too frightening a form of mental frailty for us to hold without flinching. Annihilation anxiety tends to be part of the DNA of disability organisations, being pumped, unseen, into the air breathed by both staff and clients. In coming into such a precarious, frightened organism, it is essential that the consultant maintains an attitude of revelation rather than salvation (Lawrence, 2000, pp. 173–174), with their primary concern being the discovery of truth and reality rather than the proffering of conscious solutions to unconscious problems.

It is hardly surprising, given this, that organisations working with disability have a particular vulnerability to trauma (Corbett, Cottis & Lloyd, 2011). The consultation or supervision space can be one in which to consider the exact nature of the trauma impacting upon the institution. Is it *strain* (the Chinese water torture strain of daily life), *cumulative* ("the build up of small incidents into an overpowering wave of oppression" (Hopper, 2003, p. 54)), or *catastrophic*? At the heart of all three types of trauma (which can coexist or merge) is the helplessness experienced when dependency on other people, situations, or structures fails. Such traumatised systems are vulnerable to enacting Hopper's theory of incohesion: aggregation/massification, the fourth basic assumption in the unconscious life of social systems (Hopper, 2003b). Basic assumption incohesion describes a process of oscillation between states of aggregation and massification, most often occurring when a system suffers trauma, arising largely from failed dependency on people or situations. A group veers manically between being an aggregate (a collection of minimally connected people) whose members struggle with anxiety based on isolation or lack of safety, or a mass (a collection of people with minimal individuation) which is full of anxieties based largely on fear of suffocation.

Added to the vulnerability all disability organisations have to trauma, we have to consider the almost unthinkable challenge placed on its functioning by the forensic disability patient. On both an individual and an organisational level, motivations in working with intellectual disability, while complex and underscored by ambivalence, tend to be conceptualised by us as altruistic and benign. Institutions are born from an ostensible need to care, a task made easier when the recipient of institutional care can be identified more as a victim than a victimiser. Passive recipients of care feed the carer with gratitude, imbuing the institution with a clear and comforting sense of identity. There is a fantasy that is born in the conception of an institution that it has been born to house victims, with the victimisers kept safely from view outside its walls. The forensic disability patient is not who most would choose to encounter or work with. They represent a threat to institutional health and embed anxiety within the fabric of the organisation. The threat is inside rather than out, and as such provides the institution with an existential problem that most struggle to resolve.

In consulting to a residential team working with a forensic disability patient of a colleague of mine, I was struck by the extraordinary polarity of their splitting. They were a difficult group to sit with, riven as they were by anxiety at the state to which they had been reduced since their patient had entered their home, one year before. There was an almost equal division between those workers who described the patient with empathy, care, and compassion, and those who desperately wanted this dangerous man to be removed from their service. They spoke about the iniquity of other clients being neglected by them, so time-consuming was the level of supervision and monitoring demanded by this man. Our first session took on a strangely competitive edge, as when one worker voiced her feelings of compassion for the patient, this was countered by her colleague saying how evil his past acts of abuse had been. Another worker suggested that as horrible as the abusive acts had been they should be seen as eerily precise enactments of what this man's father had subjected him to as a child. "That's no excuse for hurting any child," said another worker, "He just uses what's happened to him as a way of not taking responsibility." Towards the end of this initial session I found myself struggling with rather paralysed feelings, as if gripped myself by an anxiety about taking one side over another, pleasing one group of workers while disappointing the other. Eventually I managed to comment on the concreteness of the split, as if the patient's actions had constructed a wall straight down the middle of the team, making it impossible to adopt more nuanced thoughts about their patient's history and motivations. Perhaps, I suggested, the patient may have projected his very split, concretised, and fragmented inner world into the team, making it as difficult for them as it was for him to consider any nuances of feeling or thought. In order to keep anxiety at bay things had to be either all good or all bad, just as feelings had to be either too soft or too hard. The middle ground was too frightening to inhabit.

Over time this team did manage to address their internal split, eventually moving from what Klein (1946) would term a paranoid schizoid position to a far healthier depressive position in which their patient could be viewed in a more integrated way, being made up not just of either good or either bad experiences, feelings, and behaviours, but as an amalgam of good, bad, and all that lies between.

In consulting to an organisation in the grip of incohesion processes, a binocular view is required in order to focus not just on the overall institutional defences, but also on how they may be enacted on an individual level. In working with this institution I had been reminded of Tustin's (1981) concept of individual "crustacean" and "amoeboid" personalities—a useful way of describing two types of characterological defence against annihilation anxieties. The crustacean protects the fragility of its inner self with a hard, impermeable shell, while the amoeboid defends against the terror of aloneness by seeking merger and fusion. Caught in the ebb and flow of institutional incohesion, it is difficult for individual staff members to avoid being pulled to one or the other extreme, creating the kind of splitting processes that are commonly observed within those teams working with forensic disability patients. My work with this particular team allowed a gradual shedding of these individual defences alongside a group rejection of the massified inner group responses that had driven their initial split.

Disability attracts through its generation of sympathy and evocation of empathy. It repels through attacking our sense of normality and activating our dread of our own minds becoming damaged by close contact with deficit. Ambivalence is an inevitable component of forensic disability therapy. For supervision to fulfil its aim of improving clinical practice while helping those engaged in extremely challenging and demanding work it has to be a repository to which can be brought feelings of shame, guilt, disgust, and rage without fear of retribution or judgement. Supervision aims to construct, amongst other things, a space away from the intensity of the analytic hour in which projections, aggressive attacks, transference and countertransference phenomena can be more readily examined, and where the supervisor helps the therapist re-experience and consider aspects of the analytic interface that were unable to be held in mind during the session. At times this will involve a de-acceleration of the clinical content, allowing a slow motion, frame-by-frame re-viewing of sessions in which too much happened too quickly for thought to have been cathected in the moment. At other times a speeding up process will have to be achieved in order to prevent the slow, mindless, plodding tedium of the session from being re-enacted within the supervision.

For supervision to allow the therapist a creative space away from the heat of the analytic encounter, it has to be free from the level of anxiety that is exacerbated by the intensity of the dyadic work and that can threaten to paralyse thinking and reflection. It cannot, however, be completely devoid of anxiety, as the supervisor has to hold an objective view of the levels of risk and danger held by the patient. There is a danger of both patient and supervisor being lulled by the patient's characterological defences into a dissociative denial of the severity of his pathology. The supervisor has also to remain healthily anxious about the therapist's vulnerability to being drawn into a form of *folie à deux*, a response to the power of the forensic patient's ability to evacuate their pathology outwards. If the supervisor is not attentive to the risk of the therapist being seduced into boundary blurring or breaking, it is almost inevitable that the supervision itself becomes drawn into a perverse enactment in which thinking gets replaced by action. Boundary is all.

Forensic disability therapy is all too often a fragile being, vulnerable to envious attacks from without and fear-laden aggression from within. Supervision has to help create and maintain a protective carapace around the therapeutic work, enabling the analytic exchange to proceed without fear of attack and sabotage. The lack of societal value accorded to people with disabilities is echoed in the various ways in which systems conspire to rob disability therapy of the elements it needs in order to fulfil its potential—most prominently confidentiality, a key element of the analytic boundary. An understanding of the dynamics of the disabled organisation is required when consulting to representatives of an institution or, indeed, to the institution itself. The valency of the organisation to traumatogenic modes of functioning creates obstacles in the way of non-disabled thinking and clear communication, placing a responsibility on the supervisor or the consultant to retain their ability to think and speak without an over-identification with either trauma or disability. Splitting as a defence against both phenomena is invariably encountered in the supervisory exchanges, and can, without careful handling, become embedded within the supervisor himself, preventing the creation of new, non-disabled ways of thinking, symbolically aborting the chance of non-disabled life.

CHAPTER NINE

On saying I don't know: expedient disabilities and mind envy

Estela Welldon, the mother of contemporary forensic psychotherapy, wrote that, "When working with criminals and deviants the therapeutic task is to facilitate a movement towards acting less and suffering more, whereas with neurotics, it is to suffer less and act more" (1984, p. 108). These words have resonated throughout the writing of this book, conveying the agonising dilemma of every forensic patient: why should I want to suffer more? This is the question that is writ large in every encounter with a forensic disability patient, as we are requiring of them a commitment to give up various defence mechanisms in order to ensure that other people are kept safe. The therapeutic transformation of actions into words rarely happens smoothly, as the forensic patient has a desperate need to keep hold of their symptomology. It has in many cases become a perverse attachment object, the world of sexual aggression becoming the only secure base they can imagine having. In working with forensic disability patients we are asking them to give up aspects of their disability too.

* * *

"Matthew" is approaching his twentieth session of individual therapy. He is twenty-four, has a mild intellectual disability, and has been referred because of a series of sexual assaults on other men with disabilities, both in the community and in his group home. He is a patient who evokes warmth in many of those who care for him, despite the severity of his crimes, and I find myself experiencing some of that amiability myself. He has a friendly, engaging smile, and a childlike openness about him that invites care and concern from me. It is hard not to remark in supervision upon the deeply paternal emotions he arouses in me, and my supervisor has often had to remind me not to forget that this is a man who has perpetrated terrible abuses on others and is capable of doing so again. In thinking of him in the context of real and false self-functioning (Winnicott, 1965b), there is an ever present risk of me being seduced by the alluring false self he brings to his sessions. I hear my supervisor's words, but still somehow manage to lose touch with her concern when faced with Matthew's wide-eyed naivety in the consulting room. He enters the room looking worried and I comment on this, on how differently he looks from his usual light, bright-eyed entrance. "Something bad happened," he begins, before sitting on the chair opposite me, his hands pressed tightly together, his fingers being rubbed feverishly by him, like worry beads. I say how sorry I am to hear this, but glad he is able to tell me more about what has happened.

"Carlos says I touched his bits. I didn't touch his bits. I didn't touch any bits." He bites his hand with a quick, savage violence and draws blood, betraying an anxiety I have not seen since our first session together. "I can see how horrible you are feeling," I say. "You're safe here. You can let me know everything that happened." He nods, and rocks from side to side. The sounds of the outside world retreat, and I find myself terribly aware of the anxiety seeping out of him, like blood from a wound. I notice too that my countertransference response has altered somewhat, with much of the warmth replaced by something cooler, as I have been reminded of his potential for harm. He stammers out his words, his body shaking and his hands continually drawn to his mouth, where he gives himself little bites, like an animal nipping at his skin. He gradually tells me how the previous day he had been out for a trip to the cinema with six men and women from his day centre, accompanied by three members of staff. Halfway through the film Carlos, who was sitting next to him, punched his arm and started to shout. Both men were taken out of the auditorium by a member of staff, where Carlos alleged that Matthew had touched his genitals. The two men were taken back to their respective homes, with Matthew then being interviewed by the manager of his house. It was not yet known whether Carlos wished to press criminal charges against him.

The outline of the narrative now shared, I begin to try to investigate the details of what happened and why. He repeats, "I don't know," to every one of my questions. It gets to the point where the words are hardly out of my mouth before Matthew repeats, "I don't know," as if it has become a reflex response, a non-thinking reply that serves to stop the emergence of any further narrative. I try various interpretations—"It's hard for you to know," and, "Maybe you don't want me to know,"—but nothing intrudes upon his mantra, which has assumed the qualities of a self-soothing chant, Matthew's desperate attempt to calm the anxieties threatening to overwhelm him. He is, more than ever before, a terrified child wanting the torture to end. As the session comes to a close, we are no closer to a shared understanding of what transpired between him and Carlos, and I say, "I'll see you next week. We can carry on thinking then about all that's happened." Suddenly he looks furious and I see how quickly he can drop his facade of childlike innocence. "*You* think!" he says, his face pinched in anger. "I can't think no more." With that, he leaves the room. I notice how shaken up I feel by this last exchange, as if his words were a physical slap to my face. I try to gather myself, but his words stay with me over the next few days. I find myself wondering whether this exchange on the cusp of the session was my first glimpse of Matthew's real self, an indicator of how much false self-functioning I had been witness to over the course of our work.

Another question I am left with between this session and the next is what Matthew means when he says "I don't know". There are several possible narratives suggested by these words: that nothing happened and he is the victim of a malicious false accusation; that he cannot know about attacking Carlos because it has not occurred; or that it took place but he has had to dissociate from the event, to shield himself from having to face his compulsion to abuse. Matthew's "I don't know" may be his way of not letting me know, a more conscious attempt to evade responsibility for his abusive actions. In order to work out this conundrum, to know something more about not knowing, I try to locate it within one of a number of defensive mechanisms, some of which are unconscious, some conscious.

* * *

Sinason has written of various forms of secondary disability (Sinason, 1992), those defensive reactions overlaid on a primary cognitive deficit. The first, the mild secondary handicap, involves an exaggeration of the original disability in order to placate the outside world. This links with Bybee and Zigler's (1999) notion of "outer-directedness", in which the person with a disability adopts an overly passive and compliant persona in order to feel approved of by others. In this, the patient may have erected a protective membrane of stupefaction, an unconscious dumbing down in order to meet society's need for people with disabilities to be happy and smiling, to not allow us to be troubled by any of the misery that living with a disability can bring. When faced with questions requiring a yes/no response, people with intellectual disabilities are far more likely than their non-disabled peers to display compliance and passivity by answering "yes" (Milne, Clare & Bull, 2002), such is the unconscious terror of voicing one's own subjective truth. To say "no" is to draw attention to oneself, to reveal a self that is sustained by a harsh superego and a depleted ego. It is also to invoke disapproval, to invite the world to show its disdain.

Sinason's second secondary disability is the "opportunist handicap", a severe personality mal-development in which all internal disturbance amalgamates. The third type of secondary handicap is disability as a defence against trauma,"where the handicap is used in the service of the self to protect it from unbearable memory of trauma, of a breakdown in the protective shield" (1992, p. 23). My question of Matthew was whether his not knowing belonged in the conscious or the unconscious domains. If it was a more conscious process it fitted with what I came to think of as an expedient secondary disability. Whereas Sinason's secondary disabilities are clearly unconscious in motivation and structure, the expedient secondary disability is used *consciously* by forensic patients in order to diminish their responsibility for their actions. The patient can "not know" about why they have a disability because they cannot bear for it to be known. Their secondary handicap against trauma protects them unconsciously from the pain of having to think about how their brain was starved of oxygen at birth, or how they were screamed at as a baby, or how they are the result of "deathmaking" sex (Wolfensberger, 1987) or sex gone wrong. They can "not know" why they abused someone because they cannot bear to know that in abusing someone else they were replaying their own abuse. These are both unconscious ways of not knowing that are defensive in motivation.

The patient may say "I don't know" not because of the psychological agony of something becoming known, but because of the consequences that will befall them. They are making a conscious, intentional decision to limit access to truth because of their fear of punishment. Conscious and unconscious motivations can interweave around each other, making it extremely difficult for the clinician to differentiate unconscious from conscious secondary disabilities, as they can appear to stem from the same defensive source. What Matthew overlaid on this at the end of his session was an uncharacteristic slap of rage, a glimpse of real-self functioning that betrayed the tremendous psychic strain he had been exerting on keeping his defences so securely in place. His words, "*You* think! I can't think no more," conveyed his fury at my adopting of the role of interrogator in our session, probing him like a policeman rather than treating him like a therapist. It also raised a question about his relationship to his own disabled mind, and mine.

One of the central purposes of forensic disability therapy is to assess how much of a mind a patient has. How disabled has it been by environmental and genetic events? How capable is it of change? How able is it to hold a theory of mind, to imagine that another can have a thought or a feeling that is different from one's own? The coming together of a therapist and a patient is a meeting of minds that hold subjective differences. Within the intersubjective space of the countertransference can exist an ongoing curiosity about what it would be like to have the other's mind. For the therapist this can often be a benign form of daydreaming. I can find myself in the consulting room wondering what my life would be like if I couldn't read or write, work out numbers, or hold interesting ideas in my head. Sitting opposite the patient for whom these basic achievements are unattainable I can feel a profound sense of relief, a response that has to be checked if it is not to translate into a patronising infantilisation of the poor, wounded patient.

Daydreaming about the imagined patient without their deficits is an important aspect of the work as it represents a creative response to the trauma of disability. In "creative writers and day dreaming" (1908e) Freud contextualised daydreaming as an adult form of play, linking it with the pleasure gained from ordering the world in ways that give comfort and satisfaction. My daydreams about patients without disabilities allow the presence of something hopeful to be held in mind within the consulting room, or, indeed, outside it. Whether the phantasy is constructed mainly by me as a form of comfort against the pain of disability, or projected into me by the patient, desperate for a non-traumatising aspect of their selves to be thought about, the daydreams can help create an intersubjective space in which hope rather than despair can be maintained.

What, though, of the patient's daydreams and phantasies about *my* mind? Does he allow himself vengeful hopes that it can be as disabled, fragile, and vulnerable as his own? Or does he have instead to deal with the more painful realisation that, despite its various human vulnerabilities, its disabilities are far smaller than his? I can sometimes forget things, get confused, or lose the thread of what I am saying, but I hope I will never know, with the profound certainty that my patients know, the reality of a mind that leaks more than it can hold. The patient's response to this painful reality, that I have a mind that can do so much more than his mind, may be rooted in a deep and powerful form of envy.

Klein formulated a notion of envy that stems from "the angry feeling that another person possesses and enjoys something desirable—the envious impulse being to take it away or to spoil it" (1975, p. 176). Envy leads the child to phantasise about entering the primal good object (in Kleinian terms the good breast) and debase it specifically because it is good. The good object is then internalised, becoming part of the child's ego, causing a reversal of the prenatal state as the mother is now inside the infant. For Klein, envy is an expression of innate destructive impulses, something that is resistant to change. In his "Three contributions to the theory of sex" Freud (1908c) introduced the notion of penis envy, the girl's reaction during her psychosexual development to the realisation that she does not have a penis. Freud's declaration of this phenomenon as a crucial moment in the formation of gender and sexual identity for women has evoked much dissent, leading in part to Karen Horney's counter-theory of womb envy (Horney, 1942). She proposed that men experience womb envy more powerfully than women experience penis envy, though, unlike Freud's drive theory of penis envy as an innate trait, she placed it in a cultural, psychosocial context. I wish here to introduce the notion of *mind envy*, as a way of understanding part of Matthew's need to declare that his mind had reached its limits, and that mine would have to take its place.

One of the most painful areas the forensic disability patient has to work on is the acknowledgement of his own disability. And nowhere is this experienced more painfully than in the intensity of the transference where a yearning for fusion, blending, and synthesis falls apart in the disparity between the disabled and the non-disabled minds.

There will always be something that one cannot understand about the other—what it is like to have, on the one hand, a thinking mind and, on the other, a non-thinking mind. The forensic disability patient's object of envy, the non-disabled mind, is not the good object but the omnipotent-idealised object, thought to have qualities felt by the patient to be unattainable. As Feldman and De Paola (1994) state in their examination of early processes of envy in the infant, "The newborn's mind is overwhelmed with a sense of loss that cannot be mourned" (p. 127). Mind envy is an attempt to describe the patient's agonising yearning for what is inside the therapist's head. The disability transference is, in part, borne from the patient's projective rage at their inability to introject the therapist's mind, their need to project all of their non-thinking into the mind of the therapist, making the therapist/patient dyad symbiotic disabled twins.

The disability patient's envy of the mind that has not been disabled is not restricted to the forensic field. It manifests itself in a wider range of clinical interactions, constituting one of the most agonising dilemmas for the patient with disabilities: how to live with a malfunctioning mind and how to use the functioning mind of another. One of the aims of psychotherapeutic work is to facilitate the introjection of something good from the therapist, be that empathic feelings, the capacity to think, or the ability to regulate overwhelming feelings of loss, anxiety or rage. This tends not to happen without an intrapsychic struggle. For the patient to be able to introject a good object he has to face the painful acknowledgement that his mind is less than the mind of another. This loss is hard to grieve without rage being processed too. The patient has to struggle with feeling that another possesses and is withholding a non-disabled mind from him. This feeling of failed gratification is experienced, in Kleinian terms, as the breast withholding or keeping for itself the object of desire, leading to the kind of explosive rage leaking out from Matthew's defences. I came to think that he did consciously know that he had abused Carlos, and he was employing an expedient secondary disability to withhold this knowledge from me. His capacity to withhold was strengthened by his rage at me for having a mind that he craved. Unsurprisingly, my work with him then entered new territory, in which our joint idealisation of each other was abandoned in favour of a more explicit, and more real, negative transference containing Matthew's primitive mind envy. He could at last show his rage at me for having a mind that worked so much more effectively than his, and in the showing of this rage he was able to show me the aggression, hatred, and rage that powered so many of his sexual attacks. Unless recognised and worked with (primarily in the transference) mind envy can lead to a therapeutic impasse in which the therapist can *only* be experienced as withholding, the punitive embodiment of early experiences of maternal or paternal neglect, or, in the most severe cases, abuse.

It is not, of course, just in the area of the mind that we find differences that divide the life experience of the patient from the therapist. For the forensic disability patient, if something of the therapist's mind cannot yet be introjected there is a residual unconscious hope that less difference lies in the area of sexual perversion. This tends to be explored by the patient through the testing of therapeutic boundary. When the patient tests our boundaries he is not simply trying to squeeze an extra five minutes from us, or wanting us to let slip our marital status or what car we drive. He is probing for any holes in our protective membrane, any weak spots in the wall dividing us from him. His desire is that he is not alone in his perversion and that we can share in his abusive desires. Any deviance in the boundary can be experienced by the forensic disability patient as proof that we care as little as he does about the need for boundary. In disclosing the horrific details of his own abuse or of his abuse of others, the patient is vigilant for any signs of arousal or prurient interest in our responses, saturating the transference with an expectation that the only way he can be understood is by a mind that perversely mirrors his own. Mind envy has thus been responded to with a destructive blurring of difference, a phantasy that even if the therapist retains and withholds his non-disabled mind from the patient, they can both share a perverse mind.

These kind of therapeutic challenges are enormously painful to work through, for both patient and therapist. Forensic disability therapy is, as Welldon reminds us, often about suffering more, and I think that this suffering is at its most intense when working at the very limits of deficit and disability. Why, then, do it? The simple answer is because it works. While recent research into the treatment of forensic disability patients has tended to be limited to cognitive behavioural approaches (Michie & Lindsay, 2012; Rose, Rose, Hawkins & Anderson, 2012; Heaton & Murphy, 2013), earlier research has demonstrated the efficacy of psychodynamic and psychoanalytic treatments (Beail, 2001; Proctor & Beail, 2007). The current lack of interest in funding and conducting research into forensic approaches that differ from a broadly cognitive behavioural therapy (CBT) model is of profound concern, mirroring as it does a systemic transfer of interest from the complex, gradual, and time-consuming examination of the unconscious motivations of forensic patients to shorter, less complex, and more manualisable approaches. Both interventions, CBT and psychoanalytic (and those that lie between the two), have their benefits, with some patients being more or less suited to one or the other. It has been my experience that the level of trauma experienced and presented by forensic disability patients will more often require a therapeutic approach that can allow time in which therapist and patient can navigate and work through the blocks to healthy sexual identity that have plagued the patient. In this, I am reminded of how Anne Alvarez (2012) stresses the need for time to be taken when working with patients with autism and other disabilities by recalling the words of the art critic Robert Hughes: "What we need more of is slow art: art that holds time as a vase holds water; art that grows out of modes of perception and making, whose skill and doggedness make you think and feel; art that isn't merely sensational, that doesn't get its message across in seconds, that isn't falsely iconic, that hooks onto something deep-running in our nature" (2012, p. 20).

Intelligence is revered in our culture as much as sexual perversion is abhorred. These twinned responses consign our patients to the outmost reaches of society. Throughout this book I have attempted to bring together the disciplines of forensic psychotherapy and disability therapy in order to create a more thoughtful response which can provide some understanding of the motivations of our patients without minimising the horror of their actions. Forensic disability therapy is a discipline that involves a connection with the twin agonies felt by our patients: the constraints of living with a cognitive deficit alongside the compulsion to abuse. It also requires a capacity to contain the many potentially overwhelming aspects of disability that cause non-thinking in both our patients and ourselves.

Forensic disability therapy is an intersubjective process that involves the meeting of two minds and the creation of an intersubjective field in which differences can be tolerated, thought about, and made sense of. The key difference is that of ability—one mind is disabled and the other is not. The mutative power of therapy should allow the seemingly non-disabled mind to recognise its disabled parts and the disabled mind to become more open to thought and reflection. Western societies are structured to defend against the seemingly unthinkable thought that disability is part of us all and, as such, the *them* (disabled, damaged, wrong) and *us* (able, perfect, right) dichotomy is a meaningless fiction (Corbett, 2012). Forensic disability therapy challenges us to consider different notions of where one (non-disabled) mind ends and another (disabled) mind begins. It also has to allow us to consider where one perversion ends and another begins.

In considering the development of forensic disability therapy from its origins in forensic psychotherapy and disability therapy, one becomes aware of all that has not been able to be said as much as all that has. While my clinical orientation is psychoanalytic I hope that I have said enough about the need for forensic disability therapy to encompass more than one mode of thought. The most important aspect of this work is its capacity to be relational, for we tend to work with patients whose problems with relating have caused them to be a danger to themselves and to others. Wherever and however we have been trained as psychotherapists, we have the ability to provide the framework of a relationship that is of most use to the people with whom we work. Forensic disability patients act out, in part, as a defence against the seeming impossibility of intimacy. By providing a therapeutic space in which healthy intimacy can be explored we are attempting to disprove the patient's theory that intimacy has either to be withdrawn from or attacked.

I wrote this book in order to make sense of my learning over the past twenty years, and to gather together ideas developed along the way that could now be presented as theories to be tested and adapted by others. Although many of these ideas have shifted and changed in the process of being put into words, I remain more convinced than ever of the critical place of the countertransference in this work. Just as the characteristics of every patient population are projected into those organisations and individuals working with them, forensic disability therapy involves a complex intersubjective exchange between clinician and patient. Our clinical encounters with perversion, aggression, and broken minds make us vulnerable to becoming disabled and to enacting rather than thinking. Concepts such as the disability transference, the disabled organisation and mind envy are attempts to conceptualise transference phenomena so that we can think about feelings that are often experienced too rawly in the consulting room to be properly understood.

The writing of this book has taken place against a backdrop of savage cuts being made in services for the patients I have described. Times of recession result in an even harsher than normal relegation of the treatment needs of forensic disability patients. Our patients do not have the luxury of being hated for only one reason. They are hated because of their disability and their perversion. I suggest they are also hated because they do not conform to the requirements of the modern clinical world. The level of trauma they both experience and perpetrate means they are unsuitable for the short-term treatment models being rolled out internationally and, in the absence of the kind of in-depth, long-term psychological services they require, they tend to end up in one form of prison or another—either prison itself or a socially constructed version of it. While the damaging impact of this upon the patients themselves is inarguable, I fear that we have ignored the impact upon those whom we ask to police them. The scarcity of specialist residential units for forensic disability patients has resulted in mainstream units becoming forensic by default, with staff being expected to supervise, monitor, and, in some cases, treat the most concerning patients in the community.

I have tried to stress as democratically as possible the needs of patients, carers, families, and institutions, knowing how possible it is for the forensic burden to be felt most keenly by those paid and unpaid carers. Despite how often I have stressed the complexity and the challenge of being a forensic disability therapist, it is as nothing compared to being a forensic disability patient or someone caring for him. While psychotherapy provides a space in which the forensic burden can be passed over to another, come the end of the session it has to be handed back. I see forensic disability therapy as just one part of a wider system of support that can relieve patients and their carers of the intolerable threat of action replacing thought. Systemic collaboration has to be the default position for any service response to the forensic patient. With this in mind, I hope that some of the ideas raised in this book can help inform future trainings for clinicians and carers alike, as the paucity of forums in which creative thinking can take place is a worrying reflection of the handicapped way in which disability is currently thought about.

Just as it takes a village to raise a child, forensic disability therapy is the product of many grandparents, parents, uncles, and aunts. I think of it as being predominantly the offspring of a marriage between forensic psychotherapy and disability therapy, and, in developmental terms, of it beginning to make its first steps into the world. It still has its vulnerabilities, just as do so many forms of in-depth psychotherapy in our increasingly short-term, manualised world, but there is hope. The past two decades have seen the birth and growth of organisations such as Respond in London, Disability Psychotherapy Ireland in Dublin, and the UK and Irish Institute for Psychotherapy and Disability. All of these organisations have been strikingly inclusive in their desire to develop forensic thinking alongside the pioneering of mainstream psychotherapy for people with intellectual disabilities. Perhaps there is something in working with the trauma of disability that stops us from taking too split a view of our forensic patients. The disability therapy world has been more able than most to rise to the challenge of not creating an artificial divide between the good and the bad, and has been able to acknowledge and work with the victim in the victimiser and vice versa. This bodes well for the future of psychotherapy with people with intellectual disabilities in general, and, more specifically, for the continuing growth and resilience of forensic psychotherapy with children and adults with intellectual disabilities.

REFERENCES

Abraham, Karl (1924a). Letter to Sigmund Freud. 25th May. In: Sigmund Freud & Karl Abraham (2009). *Briefwechsel 1907–1925: Vollständige Ausgabe. Band 2: 1915–1925*. Ernst Falzeder & Ludger M. Hermanns (Eds.), pp. 765–766. Vienna: Verlag Turia und Kant.

Abraham, Karl (1924b). Letter to Sigmund Freud. 25th May. In Sigmund Freud & Karl Abraham (2002). *The Complete Correspondence of Sigmund Freud & Karl Abraham: 1907–1925. Completed Edition*. Ernst Falzeder (Ed.). Caroline Schwarzacher, Christine Trollope, & Klara Majthényi King (Transls.), pp. 505–506. London: Karnac.

Alexander, Franz, and Staub, Hugo (1929). *Der Verbrecher und seine Richter: Ein psychoanalytischer Einblick in die Welt der Paragraphen*. Vienna: Internationaler Psychoanalytischer Verlag.

Alvarez, A. (2003). Reflections on the supervision of psychotherapy with young abused/abusers. In: J. Woods (Ed.), *Boys Who Have Abused: Psychoanalytic Psychotherapy with Victim/Perpetrators of Sexual Abuse* (pp. 208–218). London and Philadelphia: Jessica Kingsley.

Alvarez, A. (2012). *The Thinking Heart: Three Levels of Psychoanalytic Therapy with Disturbed Children*. London: Routledge.

Anonymous (1926). Indian Psycho-Analytical Society: Annual Report, 1925, pp. 291–293. In Max Eitingon (Ed.). *Bulletin of the International Psycho-Analytical Association. International Journal of Psycho-Analysis, 7*: 285–295.

Antebi, D. (2003). Pathways of risk: The patient, the present and the unconscious. In: R. Doctor (Ed.), *Dangerous Patients: A Psychodynamic Approach to Risk Assessment and Management* (pp. 7–20). London: Karnac.

Aragão Oliveira, R., Milliner, E., & Page, R. (2004). Psychotherapy with physically disabled patients. *Psychoanalytic Psychotherapy, 58*(4): 430–441.

Argyle, M. (2013). *Bodily Communication* (2nd edn). London: Routledge.

Ãvila, L. A., & de Macedo, C. R. M. (2012). The "impossible" group: An experience of long-term group analytic psychotherapy for autistic people. *Group Analysis, 45*(3): 310–324.

Balint, Michael (1951). On Punishing Offenders. In: George B. Wilbur, Warner Muensterberger, & Lottie M. Maury (Eds.). *Psychoanalysis and Culture: Essays in Honor of Géza Róheim*, pp. 254–279. New York: International Universities Press.

Balint, M. (1979). *The Basic Fault: Therapeutic Aspects of Regression.* Evanstown, IL: Northwestern University Press.

Balogh, R., Bretherton, K., Whibley, S., Berney, T., Graham, S., Richold, P., Worsley, C., & Firth, H. (2001). Sexual abuse in children and adolescents with intellectual disability. *Journal of Intellectual Disability Research, 45*: 194–201.

Banerji, Manmath N. (1925). The Indian Psycho-Analytical Society: Annual Report, 1924, pp. 240–242. In: Max Eitingon (Ed.). *Bulletin of the International Psycho-Analytical Association. International Journal of Psycho-Analysis, 6*: 235–245.

Barbaree, H. E., & Marshall, W. L. (2006). An introduction to the juvenile sex offender: Terms, concepts and definitions. In: H. E. Barbaree, W. L. Marshall & S. M. Hudson (Eds.), *The Juvenile Sex Offender* (pp. 1–18). New York: The Guilford Press.

Beail, N. (1998). Psychoanalytic psychotherapy with men with intellectual disabilities: A preliminary outcome study. *British Journal of Medical Psychology, 71*: 1–11.

Beail, N. (2001). Recidivism following psychodynamic psychotherapy amongst offenders with intellectual disabilities. *The British Journal of Forensic Practice, 3*(1): 33–37.

Beail, N. (2003). What works for people with mental retardation? Critical commentary on cognitive behavioral and psychodynamic psychotherapy research. *Mental Retardation, 41*(6): 468–472.

Beail, N., Kellett, S., Newman, D. W., & Warden, S. (2007). The dose-effect relationship in psychodynamic psychotherapy with people with intellectual disabilities. *Journal of Applied Research in Intellectual Disabilities, 20*(5): 448–454.

Beail, N., Warden, S., Morsley, K., & Newman, D. W. (2005). Naturalistic evaluation of the effectiveness of psychodynamic psychotherapy for people with intellectual disabilities. *Journal of Applied Research in Intellectual Disabilities, 18*: 245–251.

Becker, J. V., & Hicks, S. J. (2003). Juvenile sexual offenders: Characteristics, interventions, and policy issues. *Annals of The New York Academy of Sciences, 989*: 397–410.

Bell, A. O., (Ed.), (1977). *The Diary of Virginia Woolf: Volume 1: 1915–19*. London: Hogarth.

Bender, M. (1993). The unoffered chair: The history of therapeutic disdain towards people with a learning difficulty. *Clinical Psychology Forum, 54*: 7–12.

Berman, L. (1993). *Beyond the Smile: The Therapeutic Use of the Photograph*. London: Routledge, Chapman and Hall.

Bertin, Célia (1982). *La Dernière Bonaparte*. Paris: Librairie Académique Perrin.

Bick, E. (1968). The experience of the skin in early object-relations. *International Journal of Psychoanalysis, 49*(3): 484–486.

Bion, W. R. (1957). Differentiation of the psychotic from non-psychotic personalities. In: W. R. Bion (Ed.), *Second Thoughts: Selected Papers on Psycho-Analysis*. New York: Jason Aronson.

Bion, W. R. (1961). *Experiences in Groups and Other Papers*. London: Tavistock.

Bion, W. R., & Rickman, J. (1943). Intra-group tensions in therapy: Their study as the task of the group. *The Lancet, 242*(6274): 678–682.

Blackman, N. (2003). *Loss and Learning Disability*. London: Worth.

Bowlby, John (1944a). Forty-Four Juvenile Thieves: Their Characters and Home-Life. *International Journal of Psycho-Analysis, 25*: 19–53.

Bowlby, John (1944b). Forty-Four Juvenile Thieves: Their Characters and Home-Life (II). *International Journal of Psycho-Analysis, 25*: 107–128.

Boyd, K. K. (1996). Power imbalances and therapy. *Focus, 11*(9): 1–4.

Brenner, C. (1974). On the nature and development of affects: A unified theory. *Psychoanalytic Quarterly, 43*: 532–556.

Britton, R. (1998). Naming and containing. In: R. Britton (Ed.), *Belief and Imagination* (pp. 19–28). London: Routledge.

Brodin, J. (1999). Play in children with severe multiple disabilities: Play with toys—a review. *International Journal of Disability, Development and Education, 46*(1): 25–34.

Brown, H., Stein, J., & Turk, V. (1995). The sexual abuse of adults with learning disabilities: Report of a second two-year incidence survey. *Mental Handicap Research, 8*(1): 22–24.

Buchanan, A. (1999). Risk and dangerousness. *Psychological Medicine, 29*: 465–473.

Buckley, J. V., Newman, D. W., Kellett, S., & Beail, N. (2006). A naturalistic comparison of the effectiveness of trainee and qualified clinical psychologists. *Psychology and Psychotherapy: Theory, Research and Practice, 79*(1): 137–144.

Bybee, J., & Zigler, E. (1999). Outerdirectedness in individuals with and without mental retardation: A review. In: E. Zigler & D. Bennett-Gates (Eds.), *Personality Development in Individuals with Mental Retardation* (pp. 165–225). Cambridge: Cambridge University Press.

Catina, A., & Tschuschke, V. (1993). A summary of empirical data from the investigation of two psychoanalytic groups by means of repetory grid technique. *Group Analysis, 33*(3): 433–447.

Chadwick, Mary (1932). The Neurotic Child. In: *Proceedings of the First International Congress on Mental Hygiene: Volume Two*, pp. 447–465. New York: International Committee for Mental Hygiene.

Clark, L. Pierce., Uniker, Thomas E., Cushing, W. K., Rourke, Ethel L., & Cairns, Margaret C. (1933). *The Nature and Treatment of Amentia: Psychoanalysis and Mental Arrest in Relation to the Science of Intelligence*. Baltimore, Maryland: William Wood and Company.

Corbett, A. (1996). *Trinity of Pain: Therapeutic Responses to Offenders with Learning Disabilities Who Commit Sexual Offences*. London: Respond.

Corbett, A. (2009). Words as a second language: The psychotherapeutic challenge of severe disability. In: T. Cottis (Ed.), *Intellectual Disability, Trauma and Psychotherapy* (pp. 45–62). London: Routledge.

Corbett, A. (2011). Silk purses and sows' ears: The social and clinical exclusion of people with intellectual disabilities. *Psychodynamic Practice, 17*(3): 273–289.

Corbett, A. (2012). Life at the borders of thought. In: J. Adlam, A. Aiyegbusi, P. Kleinot, A. Motz & C. Scanlon (Eds.), *The Therapeutic Milieu Under Fire: Security and Insecurity in Forensic Mental Health* (pp. 49–62). London: Jessica Kingsley.

Corbett, A. (2014). The invisible men: Forensic group therapy with people with intellectual disabilities. In: J. Woods & A. Williams (Eds.), *Forensic Group Psychotherapy: The Portman Clinic Approach* (pp. 183–201). London: Karnac.

Corbett, A., Cottis, T., & Lloyd, L. (2011). The survival and development of a traumatised clinic for psychotherapy for people with intellectual disabilities. In: E. Hopper (Ed.), *Trauma and Organisations* (pp. 111–126). London: Karnac.

Corbett Alan, Cottis Tamsin, & Morris Stephen (1996). *Witnessing Nurturing Protesting: Therapeutic Responses to Sexual Abuse of People with Learning Disabilities*. London: David Fulton Publishers.

Cottis, T. (2009a). Love hurts: The emotional impact of intellectual disability and sexual abuse on a family. In: T. Cottis (Ed.), *Intellectual Disability, Trauma and Psychotherapy* (pp. 75–89). London: Routledge.

Cottis, Tamsin (2009b). Life Support or Intensive Care?: Endings and Outcomes in Psychotherapy for People with Intellectual Disabilities. In: Tamsin Cottis (Ed.). *Intellectual Disability, Trauma and Psychotherapy*, pp. 189–204. London: Routledge and Hove, East Sussex: Routledge.

Cottis, T. (2011). Homeward bound: The use of therapy to build a secure and creative base for traumatised children at risk of sexually harmful behaviours. Paper presented at the International Association for Forensic Psychotherapy Annual Conference, Edinburgh.

Cox, M. (1992). *Shakespeare Comes to Broadmoor: "The Actors are Come Hither": The Performance of Tragedy in a Secure Psychiatric Hospital*. London: Jessica Kingsley.

Curen, Richard (2009). "Can They See in the Door?": Issues in the Assessment and Treatment of Sex Offenders Who Have Intellectual Disabilities. In: Tamsin Cottis (Ed.). *Intellectual Disability, Trauma and Psychotherapy*, pp. 90–113. London: Routledge/Taylor and Francis Group, and Hove, East Sussex: Routledge/Taylor and Francis Group.

De Groef, J., & Heinemann, E. (Eds.), (1999). *Psychoanalysis and Mental Handicap*. London: Free Association.

Dies, R. R. (1993). Research on group psychotherapy: Overview and clinical applications. In: A. Allonso & H. I. Swiller (Eds.), *Group Therapy in Clinical Practice* (pp. 473–518). Washington, DC: American Psychiatric Press.

Doctor, R. (2003). The role of violence in perverse psychopathology. In: R. Doctor (Ed.), *Dangerous Patients: A psychodynamic approach to risk assessment and management* (pp. 107–114). London: Karnac.

Duggan, C. (1997). Assessing risk in the mentally disordered: Introduction. *British Journal of Psychiatry, 170* (suppl. 32): 1–3.

Evans, C., Carlyle, J., & Dolan, B. (1996). An overview. In: C. Cordess & M. Cox (Eds.), *Forensic Psychotherapy: Crime, Psychodynamics and the Offender Patient* (pp. 509–542). London: Jessica Kingsley.

Feldman, E., & De Paola, H. (1994). An investigation into the psychoanalytic concept of envy. *International Journal of Psychoanalysis, 75*(2): 217–234.

Fenichel, O. (1955). *On the Psychology of Boredom*. New York: W. W. Norton.

Ferenczi, Sándor (1922). *Populäre Vorträge über Psychoanalyse*. Vienna: Internationaler Psychoanalytischer Verlag.

Foulkes, S. H. (1948). *Introduction to Group Analytic Psychotherapy*. London: Heinemann.

Foulkes, S. H. (1964). *Therapeutic Group Analysis*. London: George Allen & Unwin.

Foulkes, S. H. (1975). *Group Analytic Psychotherapy: Methods and Principles*. London: Maresfield Library.

Foulkes, S. H. (1990). Access to unconscious processes in the group analytic group. In: S. H. Foulkes and M. Pines (Eds.), *Selected Papers: Psychoanalysis and Group Analysis* (pp. 209–222). London: Karnac.

Freeman, A. G. (1994). Looking through the mirror of disability. *Women & Therapy, 14*(3–4): 79–90.

Freud, S. (1905e). Fragment of an analysis of a case of hysteria. *S. E., 7*: 1–122. London: Hogarth.

Freud, S. (1908c). On the sexual theories of children. *S. E., 9*: 205–226. London: Hogarth.

Freud, S. (1908e). Creative writers and day dreaming. *S. E., 9*: 149. London: Hogarth.

Freud, S. (1912b). The dynamics of Ttansference. *S. E., 12*: 97–108. London: Hogarth.

Freud, S. (1916d). Some character-types met with in psycho-analytic work. *S. E., 14*: 309–333. London: Hogarth.

Freud, S. (1916–1917). *Introductory Lectures on Psycho-analysis. S. E., 15*. London: Hogarth.

Freud, S. (1926d). Inhibitions, symptoms and anxiety. *S. E., 20*: 77–175.

Freud, Sigmund (1931a). Geleitworte: Prof. Dr. S. Freud, Wien. In: Georg Fuchs. *Wir Zuchthäusler: Erinnerungen des Zellengefangenen Nr. 2911*, pp. x–xi. Munich: Albert Langen.

Freud, Sigmund (1931b). Letter to Georg Fuchs. n.d., pp. 199–200. In: Kurt R. Eissler (1961). A Hitherto Unnoticed Letter by Sigmund Freud. *International Journal of Psycho-Analysis, 42*: 197–204.

Friedlander, Kate (1947). The Psycho-Analytical Approach to Juvenile Delinquency: Theory. Case-Studies. Treatment. London: Kegan Paul, Trench, Trubner and Company.

Fuchs, Georg (1931). Wir Zuchthäusler: Erinnerungen des Zellengefangenen Nr. 2911. Munich: Albert Langen.

Fyson, R. (2007). Young people with learning disabilities who sexually abuse: Understanding, identifying and responding from within generic education and welfare services. In: M. Calder (Ed.), *Working With Children and Young People Who Sexually Abuse: Taking the Field Forward* (pp. 110–122). Lyme Regis: Russell House.

Gabbard, G. O., & Lester, E. P. (2003). *Boundaries and Boundary Violations in Psychoanalysis*. Arlington, VA: American Psychiatric Publishing.

Gallego, R. (2006). *White on Black*. New York: Houghton Mifflin Harcourt.

Gil, E. (2011). *Helping Abused and Traumatized Children: Integrating Directive and Nondirective Approaches*. New York: Guilford.

Gilligan, J. (1997). *Violence: Reflections on a National Epidemic*. New York: Vintage.

Glasser, M. (1979). Some aspects of the role of aggression in the perversions. In: I. Rosen (Ed.), *Sexual Deviation* (pp. 278–305). Oxford: Oxford University Press.

Glasser, M., Kolvin, I., Campbell, D., Glasser, A., Leitch, I., & Farrelly, S. (2001). Cycle of child sexual abuse: Links between being a victim and becoming a perpetrator. *British Journal of Psychiatry, 179*(6): 482–494.

Glover, Edward (1956). Psycho-Analysis and Criminology: A Political Survey. *International Journal of Psycho-Analysis, 37*: 311–317.

Goddard, H. H. (1912). *The Kallikak Family: A Study in the Heredity of Feeble-Mindedness*. New York: Macmillan.

Goldin-Meadow, S. (2006). Meeting other minds through gesture: How children use their hands to reinvent language and distribute cognition. In: N. J. Enfield & S. C. Levinson (Eds.), *Roots of Human Sociality: Culture, Cognition and Interaction* (pp. 353–374). Oxford: Berg.

Grandin, T. (2006). *Thinking in Pictures: And Other Reports From My Life With Autism*. London: Bloomsbury.

Green, V. (2000). Therapeutic space for re-creating the child in the mind of the parents. In: J. Tsiantis (Ed.), *Work With Parents: Psychoanalytic Psychotherapy With Children and Adolescents* (pp. 25–45). London: Karnac.

Greenberg, L., & Safran, J. (1984). Integrating affect and cognition: A perspective on the process of therapeutic change. *Cognitive Therapy and Research, 8*(6): 559–578.

Grove, N., Bunning, K., Porter, J., & Olsson, C. (1999). See what I mean: Interpreting the meaning of communication by people with severe and profound intellectual disabilities. *Journal of Applied Research in Intellectual Disabilities, 12*(3): 190–203.

Grzesiak, Roy C., & Hicok, Dina A. (1994). A Brief History of Psychotherapy and Physical Disability. *American Journal of Psychotherapy, 48*: 240–250.

Guilfoyle, M. (2007). Grounding a critical psychoanalysis in frameworks of power. *Theory & Psychology, 17*(4): 563–585.

Hackett, S. (2004). *What Works For Children and Young People With Harmful Sexual Behaviours?* Ilford: Barnardos.

Happel, Clara (1926). Notes on an Analysis of a Case of Paederasty. *International Journal of Psycho-Analysis, 7*: 229–236.

Hartnack, Christiane (2001). Psychoanalysis in Colonial India. New Delhi: Oxford University Press.

Heaton, K. M., & Murphy, G. H. (2013). Men with intellectual disabilities who have attended sex offender treatment groups: A follow-up. *Journal of Applied Research in Intellectual Disabilities, 26*(5): 489–500.

Hinshelwood, R. D. (1999). Countertransference. *International Journal of Psychoanalysis, 80*(4): 797–818.

Hollins, Sheila (1990a). Group Analytic Therapy with People with Mental Handicap. In: Anton Dŏsen, Adriaan van Gennep, & Gosewijn J. Zwanikken (Eds.). *Treatment of Mental Illness and Behavioral Disorder in the Mentally Retarded: Proceedings of the International Congress. May 3–4, 1990. Amsterdam, The Netherlands*, pp. 81–89. Leiden: Logon Publications.

Hollins, Sheila (1990b). Grief Therapy for People with Mental Handicap. In: Anton Dŏsen, Adriaan van Gennep, & Gosewijn J. Zwanikken (Eds.). *Treatment of Mental Illness and Behavioral Disorder in the Mentally Retarded: Proceedings of the International Congress. May 3–4, 1990. Amsterdam, The Netherlands*, pp. 139–142. Leiden: Logon Publications.

Hollins, Sheila (1997). Counselling and Psychotherapy. In: Oliver Russell (Ed.). Seminars in the Psychiatry of Learning Disabilities, pp. 245–258. London: Gaskell/Royal College of Psychiatrists.

Hollins, S., & Grimer, M. (1988). *Going Somewhere: People with Mental Handicaps and their Pastoral Care*. London: SPCK.

Hollins Sheila, & Sinason Valerie (2000). Psychotherapy, Learning Disabilities and Trauma: New Perspectives. *British Journal of Psychiatry, 176*: 32–36.

Hook, J. (2001). The role of Psychodynamic psychotherapy in a modern general psychiatry service. *Advances in Psychiatric Treatment, 7*(6): 461–468.

Hopper, E. (1991). Encapsulation as a defense against the fear of annihilation. *International Journal of Psychoanalysis, 72*(4): 607–624.

Hopper, E. (2003a). *The Social Unconscious: Selected Papers*. London: Jessica Kingsley.

Hopper, E. (2003b). *Traumatic Experience in the Unconscious Life of Groups: The Fourth Basic Assumption: incohesion:aggregation/massification or (ba) I:A/M*. London: Jessica Kingsley Publishers.

Hopper, E. (2012). *Trauma and Organizations*. London: Karnac.

Horney, K. (1942). *The Collected Works of Karen Horney*. New York: W. W. Norton.

Iacono, T., & Johnson, H. (2004). Patients with disabilities and complex communication needs: The GP consultation. *Australian Family Physician, 33*(8): 585–589.

Jones, Ernest (1936). M.D. Eder: 1866–1936. *International Journal of Psycho-Analysis, 17*: 143–146.

Jones, J. (2007). Persons with intellectual disabilities in the criminal justice system: Review of issues. *International Journal of Offender Therapy and Comparative Criminology, 51*(6): 723–733.

Kahr, Brett (2000a). The Adventures of a Psychotherapist: A New Breed of Clinicians—Disability Psychotherapists. *Psychotherapy Review, 2*: 193–194.

Kahr, Brett (2000b). Psychotherapy and Learning Disabilities. *Psychotherapy Review, 2*: 205–207.

Kahr, Brett (2000c). Towards the Creation of Disability Psychotherapists. *Psychotherapy Review, 2*: 420–423.

Kahr, Brett (2000d). The Institute of Psychotherapy and Disability. *The Psychotherapist, 14*: 18, 21.

Kahr, Brett (2001). Winnicott's Contribution to the Study of Dangerousness. In: Brett Kahr (Ed.). *Forensic Psychotherapy and Psychopathology: Winnicottian Perspectives*, pp. 1–10. London: Karnac.

Keats, J. (1817). *Letters*. Oxford: Oxford University Press.

Kelly, G., & Wadey, E. (2012). Boundaries in forensic mental health nursing: Set in stone or shifting sands? In: A. Aiyegbusi & G. Kelly (Eds.), *Professional and Therapeutic Boundaries in Forensic Mental Health Practice* (pp. 113–123). London: Jessica Kingsley.

Kennedy, H., Landor, M., & Todd, L. (Eds.), (2011). *Video Interaction Guidance: A Relationship-based Intervention to Promote Attunement, Empathy and Wellbeing*. London: Jessica Kingsley.

Keogh, T. (2011). *The Internal World of the Juvenile Sex Offender: Through a Glass Darkly Then Face to Face*. London: Karnac.

Kernberg, O. F. (1993). Paranoiagenesis in organisations. In: H. I. Kaplan & B. J. Sadock (Eds.), *Comprehensive Group Psychotherapy* (pp. 45–57). Baltimore, MD: Williams & Wilkins.

King, R. (2005). CAT, the therapeutic relationship and working with people with learning disability. *Reformulation, 24*: 10–14.

Klein, M. (1935). A contribution to the psychogenesis of manic-depressive states. In: *Love, Guilt and Reparation and Other Works 1921–1945: The Writings of Melanie Klein, Volume 1* (pp. 262–289). London: Hogarth, 1975.

Klein, M. (1946). Notes on some schizoid mechanisms. *International Journal of Psychoanalysis, 27*: 99–110.

Klein, M. (1975). *Envy and Gratitude and Other Works*. London: Hogarth.

Kohut, H. (1971). *The Analysis of the Self: A Systematic Psychoanalytic Approach to the Treatment of Narcissistic Personality Disorders*. New York: International Universities Press.

Krystal, H. (1978). Trauma and affects. *The Psychoanalytic Study of the Child, 33*: 81–116.

Kumin, I. (1985). Erotic horror: Desire and resistance in the psychoanalytic setting. *International Journal of Psychoanalytic Psychotherapy, 11*: 3–20.

Langs, R. (1994). *Doing Supervision and Being Supervised*. London: Karnac.

Lawrence, W. G. (2000). *Tongued With Fire: Groups in Experience*. London: Karnac.

Lepper, G., & Riding, N. (2006). *Researching the Psychotherapy Process: A Practical Guide to Transcript-based Methods*. Basingstoke: Palgrave Macmillan.

Levitas, A. S., & Hurley, A. D. (2007). Overmedication as a manifestation of countertransference. *Mental Health Aspects of Developmental Disabilities, 10*(2): 1–5.

Lichtman, R. (1990). Psychoanalysis: Critique of Habermas' prototype of critical social sciences. *New Ideas in Psychology, 8*(3): 357–374.

Linde, C. (1993). *Life Stories: The Creation of Coherence*. Oxford: Oxford University Press.

Lindsay, W. R. (2002). Integration of recent reviews on offenders with intellectual disabilities. *Journal of Applied Research in Intellectual Disabilities, 15*(2): 111–119.

Lindy, J. D. (1985). The trauma membrane and other clinical concepts derived from psychotherapeutic work with survivors of natural disasters. *Psychiatric Annals, 15*(3): 153–160.

Lloyd-Owen, D. (1997). From action to thought: Supervising mental health workers with forensic patients. In: B. Martindale, M. Morner, M. Eugenia, C. Rodriguez & J. -P. Vidit (Eds.), *Supervision and Its Vicissitudes* (pp. 87–100). London: Karnac.

Long, S. (2012). Trauma as cause and effect of perverse organisational process. In: E. Hopper (Ed.) *Trauma and Organizations* (pp. 45–64). London: Karnac.

Lorand, Sandor (1940). Compulsive Stealing: Contribution to the Psychopathology of Cleptomania. *Journal of Criminal Psychopathology, 1*: 247–253.

MacKinlay, L., & Langdon, P. E. (2009). Staff attributions towards men with intellectual disability who have a history of sexual offending and challenging behaviour. *Journal of Intellectual Disability Research, 53*(9): 807–815.

Mahler, M. S. (1971). A study of the separation-individuation process: And its possible application to borderline phenomena in the psychoanalytic situation. *The psychoanalytic study of the child, 26*: 403–424.

Mann, D. (1994). The psychotherapist's erotic subjectivity. *British Journal of Psychotherapy, 10*: 344–354.

Mann, D. (1999). *Erotic Narratives in Psychoanalytic Practice*. London: Routledge.

Mannoni, Maud (1964a). *L'Enfant arriéré et sa mère: Étude psychanalytique*. Paris: Éditions du Seuil.

Mannoni, Maud (1964b). *The Retarded Child and the Mother: A Psychoanalytic Study*. Alan M. Sheridan Smith (Transl.). (1973). London: Tavistock Publications.

Marks, D. (1999). *Disability: Controversial Debates and Psychosocial Perspectives By Deborah Marks*. London: Routledge.

McGauley, G., & Humphrey, M. (2003). Contribution of forensic psychotherapy to the care of forensic patients. *Advances in Psychiatric Treatment, 9*(2): 117–124.

McMahon, L. (2009). *The Handbook of Play Therapy and Therapeutic Play* (2nd edn). Hove: Routledge.

Mehrebrian, A. (1971). *Silent Messages*. Belmont, CA: Wandsworth.

Meloy, J. R. (1992). *The Psychopathic Mind: Origins, Dynamics and Treatment*. Lanham, MD: Rowman & Littlefield.

Menzies Lyth, I. (1960). A case-study in the functioning of social systems as a defence against anxiety: A report on a study of the nursing service of a general hospital. *Human Relations, 13*: 95–121.

Menzies Lyth, I. (1988). *Containing Anxiety in Institutions: Selected Essays*. London: Free Association.

Michie, A. M., & Lindsay, W. R. (2012). A treatment component designed to enhance empathy in sex offenders with an intellectual disability. *The British Journal of Forensic Practice, 14*(1): 40–48.

Miller, E. J. (1993). *Power, Authority, Dependency and Change*. London: Free Association.

Milne, R., Clare, I. C., & Bull, R. (2002). Interrogative suggestibility among witnesses with mild intellectual disabilities: The use of an adaptation of the GSS. *Journal of Applied Research in Intellectual Disabilities, 15*(1): 8–17.

Moellenhoff, Fritz (1966). Hanns Sachs: 1881–1947. The Creative Unconscious. In: Franz Alexander, Samuel Eisenstein, & Martin Grotjahn (Eds.). *Psychoanalytic Pioneers*, pp. 180–199. New York: Basic Books.

Monahan, J. (1993). Limiting therapist exposure to Tarasoff Liability: Guidelines for risk containment. *American Psychologist, 48*: 242–250.

Money-Kyrle, R. (1968). Cognitive development. *International Journal of Psychoanalysis, 49*: 691–697.

Montgomery, C. (2002). Role of dynamic group therapy in psychiatry. *Advances in Psychiatric Treatment, 8*: 34–41.

Morrison, B. (1997). *As If: A Crime, a Trial, a Question of Childhood*. London: St. Martin's.

Muller, J. F. (2011). Disability, ambivalence, and the law. *American Journal of Law & Medicine, 37*: 469–521.

Mundy, P., Kascari, C., Sigman, M., & Ruskin. (1995). Nonverbal communication and early language acquisition in children with Down syndrome and in normally developing children. *Journal of Speech and Hearing Research, 38*: 157–167.

Natterson, Joseph M. (1966). Theodor Reik: b. 1888. Masochism in Modern Man. In: Franz Alexander, Samuel Eisenstein, & Martin Grotjahn (Eds.). *Psychoanalytic Pioneers*, pp. 249–264. New York: Basic Books.

Nitsun, M. (1996). *The Anti-group: Destructive Forces in the Group and Their Creative Potential*. London: Routledge.

NSPCC (2003). *"It Doesn't Happen to Disabled Children": Child Protection and Disabled Children. Report of the National Working Group on Child Protection and Disability*. London: NSPCC.

Nunberg Herman, & Federn, Ernst (Eds.). (1962). *Minutes of the Vienna Psychoanalytic Society: Volume I: 1906–1908*. Margarethe Nunberg (Transl.). New York: International Universities Press.

Nunberg Herman, & Federn, Ernst (Eds.). (1976). *Protokolle der Wiener Psychoanalytischen Vereinigung: Band I. 1906–1908*. Frankfurt am Main: S. Fischer/S. Fischer Verlag.

O'Brien, F. (2004). The making of mess in art therapy: Attachment, trauma and the brain. *Inscape, 9*(1): 2–13.

O'Connor, K. J., & Schaefer, C. E. (Eds.), (1994). *Handbook of Play Therapy. Volume Two: Advances and Innovations*. New York: Wiley.

O'Driscoll, David (1999). *A Short History of People with Learning Difficulties*. Unpublished Typescript.

O'Driscoll, David (2000). *"The Need for a Better Understanding of the Emotional Life of the Feebleminded": Two Pioneers of Psychoanalytic Psychotherapy with People with Learning Difficulties*. M.A. in Psychotherapy and Counselling, City University, London, at School of Psychotherapy and Counselling, Regent's College, Inner Circle, Regent's Park, London.

O'Driscoll, D. (2009). Psychotherapy and intellectual disability: A historical view. In: T. Cottis (Ed.), *Intellectual Disability, Trauma and Psychotherapy* (pp. 9–28). London: Routledge.

Oberndorf, Clarence P. (1939). Voyeurism as a Crime. *Journal of Criminal Psychopathology, 1*: 103–111.

Ogden, T. H. (2005). On psychoanalytic supervision. *International Journal of Psychoanalysis, 86*(5): 1265–1280.

Olsson, M. B., & Hwang, C. P. (2001). Depression in mothers and fathers of children with intellectual disability. *Journal of Intellectual Disability Research, 45*(6): 535–543.

Orbach, S. (2003). Part I: There is no such thing as a body. *British Journal of Psychotherapy, 20*(1): 3–16.

Parker, R. (2005). *Torn in Two: The Experience of Maternal Ambivalence*. London: Virago.

Payne, Sylvia M. (1957). Dr. Ethilda Budgett-Meakin Herford. *International Journal of Psycho-Analysis, 38*: 276.

Phillips, A. (1993). *On Kissing, Tickling, and Being Bored: Psychoanalytic Essays on the Unexamined Life*. London: Faber and Faber.

Phillips, A. (2000). On translating a person. In: A. Phillips (Ed.), *Promises Promises* (pp. 125–147). London: Faber and Faber.

Piaget, J. (1960). The general problems of the psychobiological development of the child. *Discussions on Child Development, 4*: 3–27.

Piaget, J. (1964). Part I: Cognitive development in children: Piaget development and learning. *Journal of Research in Science Teaching, 2*(3): 176–186.

Piaget, J. (1981). *Intelligence and Affectivity: Their Relationship During Child Development* (Trans. & Ed. T. A. Brown & C. E. Kaegi). Palo Alto, CA: Annual Reviews.

Pierce Clark, L. (1918). A character study of the hemiplegic epileptic. *American Journal of Medical Sciences, 6*(XLV): 796.

Pierce Clark, L. (1920). A clinical study of some mental contents in epileptic attacks. *Psychoanalytic Review, 7*(4): 366–375.

Pierce Clark, L. (1926). A further contribution to the psychology of the essential epileptic. *Journal of Nervous and Mental Disease, 63*(6): 575–585.

Pierce Clark, L. (1933). *The Nature and Treatment of Amentia*. London: Baillière, Tindall & Cox.

Pines, M. (2000). *The Evolution of Group Analysis*. London: Jessica Kingsley.

Proctor, T., & Beail, N. (2007). Empathy and theory of mind in offenders with intellectual disability. *Journal of Intellectual & Developmental Disability, 32*(2): 10.

Raphael-Leff, J. (2001). *Pregnancy: The Inside Story*. London: Karnac.

Regnard, C., Reynolds, J., Watson, B., Matthews, D., Gibson, L., & Clarke, C. (2007). Understanding distress in people with severe communication difficulties: Developing and assessing the Disability Distress Assessment Tool (DisDAT). *Intellectual Disability Research, 51*: 277–292.

Reiss, S., Levitan, G. W., & Szyszko, J. (1982). Emotional disturbance and mental retardation: Diagnostic overshadowing. *American Journal of Mental Deficiency, 86*: 567–574.

Rose, J., West, C., & Clifford, D. (2000). Group interventions for anger in people with intellectual disabilities. *Research in Developmental Disabilities, 21*(3): 171–181.

Rose, J., Rose, D., Hawkins, C., & Anderson, C. (2012). A sex offender treatment group for men with intellectual disabilities in a community setting. *The British Journal of Forensic Practice, 14*(1): 21–28.

Rosenfeld, H. (1987). *Impasse and Interpretation: Therapeutic and Anti-therapeutic Factors in the Psychoanalytic Treatment of Psychotic, Borderline, and Neurotic Patients*. London: Routledge.

Ruffman, T., Slade, L., & Crowe, E. (2002). The relation between children's and mothers' mental state language and theory-of-mind understanding. *Child Development, 73*(3): 734–751.

Rustin, M. (2000). Dialogues with parents. In: J. Tsiantis (Ed.), *Work With Parents: Psychoanalytic Psychotherapy With Children and Adolescents* (pp. 1–24). London: Karnac.

Rütten, Thomas (2011). Early Modern Medicine. In: Mark Jackson (Ed.). *The Oxford Handbook of the History of Medicine*, pp. 60–81. Oxford: Oxford University Press.

Ryan, G., & Lane, S. (1997). *Juvenile Sexual Offending: Causes, Consequences and Correction*. San Francisco: Jossey-Bass.

Ryle, A., & Kerr, I. (2002). *Introducing Cognitive Analytic Therapy: Principles and Practice*. Chichester: John Wiley.

Schaafsma, D., Stoffelen, J. M. T., Kok, G., & Curfs, L. M. G. (2013). Exploring the development of existing sex education programmes for people with intellectual disabilities: An Iitervention mapping approach. *Journal of Applied Research in Intellectual Disabilities, 26*(2): 157–166.

Scheffer, J. H. (1996). The setting: General considerations. In: C. Cordess & M. Cox. (Eds.), *Forensic Psychotherapy: Crime, Psychodynamics and the Offender Patient* (pp. 385–392). London: Jessica Kingsley.

Schegloff, E. A. (1992). Repair after next turn: The last structurally provided defense of intersubjectivity in conversation. *American journal of sociology, 97*(5): 1295–1345.

Scheidlinger, S. (1982). Presidential address: On scapegoating in group psychotherapy. *International Journal of Group Psychotherapy, 32*: 131–143.

Schneider, C. E. (1998). *The Practice of Autonomy: Patients, Doctors, and Medical Decisions*. Oxford: Oxford University Press.

Segal, H. (1986a). Countertransference. In: H. Segal (Ed.), *The Work of Hanna Segal: A Kleinian Approach to Clinical Practice* (pp. 81–87). London: Free Association.

Segal, H. (1986b). The function of dreams. In: H. Segal (Ed.), *The Work of Hanna Segal: A Kleinian Approach to Clinical Practice* (pp. 89–97). London: Free Association.

Segal, J. (1996). Whose disability? Countertransference in work with people with disabilities. *Psychodynamic Counselling, 2*(2): 155–166.

Seguin, E. (1856). Origin of the treatment and training of idiots. *American Journal of Education, 2*(8): 145–152.

Servais, L. (2006). Sexual health care in persons with intellectual disabilities. *Mental Retardation and Developmental Disabilities Research Reviews, 12*(1): 48–56.

Seto, M. C., & Lalumière, M. L. (2010). What is so special about male adolescent sexual offending? A review and test of explanations through meta-analysis. *Psychological Bulletin, 136*(4): 526–575.

Simon, R. I. (1999). Therapist-patient sex: From boundary violations to sexual misconduct. *Psychiatric Clinics of North America, 22*(1): 31–47.

Sinason, V. (1986). Secondary mental handicap and its relationship to trauma. *Psychoanalytic Psychotherapy,* 2(2): 131–154.

Sinason Valerie (1990). Individual Psychoanalytical Psychotherapy with Severely and Profoundly Handicapped Patients. In: Anton Dŏsen, Adriaan van Gennep, & Gosewijn J. Zwanikken (Eds.). *Treatment of Mental Illness and Behavioral Disorder in the Mentally Retarded: Proceedings of the International Congress. May 3–4, 1990.* Amsterdam, The Netherlands, pp. 71–80. Leiden: Logon Publications.

Sinason, Valerie (1991). *A Brief and Selective Look at the History of Disability.* Unpublished Typescript.

Sinason, V. (1992). *Mental Handicap and the Human Condition: New Approaches from the Tavistock.* London: Free Association.

Sinason Valerie (1999). Psychoanalysis and Mental Handicap: Experience from the Tavistock Clinic. In: Johan De Groef & Evelyn Heinemann (Eds.). *Psychoanalysis and Mental Handicap.* Andrew Weller (Transl.), pp. 194–206. London: Free Association Books.

Sinason, Valerie (2010). *Mental Handicap and the Human Condition: An Analytic Approach to Intellectual Disability.* Revised Edition. London: Free Association Books.

Sinason, V., & Osborne, E. L. (1993). *Understanding Your Handicapped Child.* London: Rosendale Press.

Smeijsters, H., & Cleven, G. (2006). The treatment of aggression using arts therapies in forensic psychiatry: Results of a qualitative inquiry. *The Arts in Psychotherapy, 33*: 37–58.

Smith, Maurice Hamblin (1924). The Mental Conditions Found in Certain Sexual Offenders. *The Lancet.* 29th March, pp. 643–646.

Snowden, P. (1997). Practical aspects of clinical risk management. *British Journal of Psychiatry, 170*: (supplement): 32–34.

Sobsey, D. (1994). *Violence and Abuse in the Lives of People With Disabilities: The End of Silent Acceptance?* Baltimore, MD: Paul H. Brookes.

Söder, M. (1990). Prejudice or ambivalence? Attitudes toward persons with disabilities. *Disability, Handicap & Society, 5*(3): 227–241.

Solomon, J., & George, C. (2011). *Disorganization of Attachment and Caregiving: Research and Clinical Advances.* New York, NY: Guilford.

Sterland, E. (2013). Sex education: Young people with learning disabilities are being left out. *Guardian* [online]. Available at: http://www.theguardian.com/social-care-network/2013/sep/17/sex-education-young-people-learning-disabilities [Accessed March 2014].

Stoddart, K. P., Burke, L., & Temple, V. (2002). Outcome evaluation of bereavement groups for adults with intellectual disabilities. *Journal of Applied Research in Intellectual Disabilities, 15*(1): 28–35.

Stoddart, William H. B. (1923). Delinquency and Mental Defect (IV). *British Journal of Medical Psychology, 3*: 188–193.

Sullivan, H. S. (1953). *The Collected Works*. New York: Norton.

Symington, J., & Symington, N. (2002). *The Clinical Thinking of Wilfred Bion*. London: Routledge.

Symington, N. (1992). Countertransference with mentally handicapped clients. In: A. Waitman & S. Conboy-Hill (Eds.), *Psychotherapy and Mental Handicap* (pp. 132–138). London: Sage.

Talbot, T. J., & Langdon, P. E. (2006). A revised sexual knowledge assessment tool for people with intellectual disabilities: is sexual knowledge related to sexual offending behaviour? *Journal of Intellectual Disability Research, 50*(7): 523–531.

Temple, N. (1996). Transference and countertransference: General and forensic aspects. In: C. Cordess & M. Cox (Eds.), *Forensic Psychotherapy: Crime, Psychodynamics and the Offender Patient: Volume 1* (pp. 23–41). London: Jessica Kingsley.

Tustin, F. (1981). *Autistic States in Children*. London: Routledge & Kegan Paul.

Van Velson, C. (2010). Psychotherapeutic understanding and approach to psychosis in mentally disordered offenders. In: A. Bartlett & G. McGauley (Eds.), *Forensic Mental Health: Concepts, Systems, Practice* (pp. 163–178). Oxford: Oxford University Press.

Varughese, S. J., & Luty, J. (2010). Stigmatised attitudes towards intellectual disability: A randomised crossover trial. *The Psychiatrist, 34*(8): 318–322.

Veneziano, C., & Veneziano, L. (2002). Adolescent sex offenders: A review of the literature. *Trauma, Violence, & Abuse, 3*(4): 247–260.

Villa, A. (2013). *Psychoanalysis and Severe Handicap: The Hand in the Cap*. London: Karnac.

Vizard, E., Monck, E., & Misch, P. (1995). Child and adolescent sex abuse perpetrators: A review of the research literature. *Journal of Child Psychology and Psychiatry, 36*(5): 731–756.

von Winterstein, Alfred Freiherr (1912). Zur Psychoanalyse des Reisens. *Imago, 1*: 489–506.

Waitman, A., & Conboy-Hill, S. (Eds.), (1992). *Psychotherapy and Mental Handicap*. London, Sage.

Wangh, M. (1975). Boredom in psychoanalytic perspective. *Social Research, 42*: 538–550.

Watermeyer, B. (2012). Disability and countertransference in group psychotherapy: Connecting social oppression with the clinical frame. *International Journal of Group Psychotherapy, 62*(3): 392–417.

Weigert, E. (1967). Narcissism: Benign and malignant forms. In: R. W. Gibson (Ed.), *Crosscurrents in Psychiatry and Psychoanalysis* (pp. 222–228). Philadelphia, PA: Lippincott.

Welldon, E. V. (1984). Application of group psychotherapy to those with sexual perversions. In: T. E. Lear (Ed.), *Spheres of Group Analysis* (pp. 9–26). London: Leinster Leader.

Welldon, E. V. (1996a). Contrasts in male and female sexual perversions. In: C. Cordess & M. Cox (Eds.), *Forensic Psychotherapy: Crime, Psychodynamics and the Offender Patient: Volume 2* (pp. 273–289). London: Jessica Kingsley.

Welldon, E. V. (1996b). Group-analytic psychotherapy in an out-patient setting. In: C. Cordess and M. Cox (Eds.), *Forensic Psychotherapy: Crime, Psychodynamics and the Offender Patient* (pp. 63–82). London: Jessica Kingsley.

Welldon, E. V. (1997). Let the treatment fit the crime: Forensic group psychotherapy. *Group Analysis, 30*: 9–26.

Welldon, E. V. (2011). *Playing with Dynamite: A Personal Approach to the Psychoanalytic Understanding of Perversions, Violence, and Criminality*. London: Karnac.

Wilber, K. (1984). The developmental spectrum and psychopathology: II. Treatment modalities. *Journal of Transpersonal Psychology, 16*(2): 137–166.

Wilkinson, M. (2006). *Coming Into Mind*. London: Taylor & Francis.

Wilson, J. P., Lindy, J. D., & Raphael, B. (1994). Empathic strain and therapist defense: Type I and II CTRs. In: J. P. Wilson & J. D. Lindy (Eds.), *Countertransference in the Treatment of PTSD* (pp. 31–61). London: The Guilford Press.

Wilson, Shula (2003). *Disability, Counselling and Psychotherapy: Challenges and Opportunities*. Houndmills, Basingstoke, Hampshire: Palgrave Macmillan.

Winnicott, Donald W. (1935). The manic defence. In: Donald W. Winnicott (1958). *Collected Papers: Through Paediatrics to Psycho-Analysis*, pp. 129–144. London: Tavistock Publications.

Winnicott, Donald W. (1943). Delinquency research. *New Era in Home and School, 24*: 65–67.

Winnicott, D. W. (1949). Hate in the counter-transference. *International Journal of Psychoanalysis, 30*: 69–74.

Winnicott, Donald W. (1956). The antisocial tendency. In: Donald W. Winnicott (1958). *Collected Papers: Through Paediatrics to Psycho-Analysis*, pp. 306–315. London: Tavistock Publications.

Winnicott, Donald W. (1958). Dr. Ambrose Cyril Wilson. *International Journal of Psycho-Analysis, 39*: 617.

Winnicott, Donald W. (1962–1963). The Antisocial Tendency Illustrated by a Case. *A Criança Portuguesa, 21*: 195–209.

Winnicott, D. W. (1964). Further thoughts on babies as persons. In: *The Child, the Family, and the Outside World* (pp. 85–92). Harmondsworth: Penguin.

Winnicott, D. W. (1965a). Ego distortion in terms of true and false self. In: M. Khan (Ed.), *The Maturational Process and the Facilitating Environment: Studies in the Theory of Emotional Development* (pp. 140–152). New York: International University Press.

Winnicott, D. W. (1965b). *The Maturational Processes and the Facilitating Environment: Studies in the Theory of Emotional Development. International Psycho-Analytical Library*. London: Hogarth.

Winnicott, Donald W. (1966). A Psychoanalytic View of the Antisocial Tendency. In: Ralph Slovenko (Ed.). *Crime, Law and Corrections*, pp. 102–130. Springfield, Illinois: Charles C. Thomas, Publisher.

Winnicott, Donald W. (1968). Delinquency as a Sign of Hope. *Prison Service Journal, 7, Number 27*: 2–7.

Winnicott, Donald W. (1984). *Deprivation and Delinquency*. Clare Winnicott, Ray Shepherd, & Madeleine Davis (Eds.). London: Tavistock Publications.

Winnicott, Donald W. (n.d.). *Meet to Be Stolen From*. Typescript. PP/DWW/A/A/2. Donald Woods Winnicott Collection. Contemporary Medical Archives Centre, Archives and Manuscripts, Rare Materials Room, The Wellcome Library for the History and Understanding of Medicine, Wellcome Collection, The Wellcome Building, London.

Wolfensberger, W. (1987). *The New Genocide of Handicapped and Afflicted People*. New York: Syracuse.

Woods, J. (2003). *Boys Who Have Abused: Psychoanalytic Psychotherapy with Victims/Perpetrators of Sexual Abuse*. London: Jessica Kingsley.

Wrye, H. K., & Welles, J. K. (2013). *The Narration of Desire: Erotic Transferences and Countertransferences*. London: Routledge.

Xenitidis, K. I., Barnes, J., & White, J. (2005). Forensic psychotherapy for adults with learning disabilities: An inpatient group-analytic group. *Group Analysis, 38*(3): 427–438.

Yalom, I. D. (1970). *The Theory and Practice of Group Psychotherapy*. New York: Basic.

INDEX